Refle....   ing

Reflective Practice in Nursing

Third Edition

Edited by

Chris Bulman
MSc, BSc (Hons), RGN, RNT, PGCEA
Senior Lecturer, School of Health and Social Care,
Oxford Brookes University

Sue Schutz
MSc, RGN, Cert Ed (FE)
Senior Lecturer, School of Health and Social Care,
Oxford Brookes University

Blackwell
Publishing

Editorial offices:
Blackwell Publishing Ltd, 9600 Garsington Road, Oxford OX4 2DQ, UK
  Tel: +44 (0)1865 776868
Blackwell Publishing Inc., 350 Main Street, Malden, MA 02148-5020, USA
  Tel: +1 781 388 8250
Blackwell Publishing Asia Pty Ltd, 550 Swanston Street, Carlton, Victoria 3053, Australia
  Tel: +61 (0)3 8359 1011

First edition published 1994 by Blackwell Publishing Ltd
Reprinted 1994, 1995 (twice), 1996 (twice), 1997
Second edition published 2000
Reprinted 2001 (twice), 2003
Third edition published 2004
Reprinted 2005

Library of Congress Cataloging-in-Publication Data is available

ISBN-10: 1-4051-1112-7
ISBN-13: 978-14051-1112-6

A catalogue record for this title is available from the British Library

Set in 10/12 pt Berkeley
by DP Photosetting, Aylesbury, Bucks
Printed and bound in Great Britain
by MPG Books Ltd, Bodmin, Cornwall

For further information on Blackwell Publishing, visit our website:
www.blackwellpublishing.com

To our students and colleagues, past and present

Contents

List of Contributors

Carrie Angove MSc, BSc (Hons), RGN, RNT, PGDE, ONC, Senior Lecturer, School of Health and Social Care, Oxford Brookes University.

Sue Atkins MSc, RN, RM, DipN Ed, Principal Lecturer, School of Health and Social Care, Oxford Brookes University.

Chris Bulman MSc, BSc (Hons), RGN, RNT, PGCEA, Senior Lecturer, School of Health and Social Care, Oxford Brookes University.

Sue Duke MSc, BSc (Hons), RGN, RNT, ONC, PG Dip, Nurse Consultant/Principal Lecturer, Royal Berkshire and Battle Hospitals NHS Trust, Reading and Oxford Brookes University.

Melanie Jasper PhD, MSc, BNurs, BA, RGN, RM, RHV, NDNCert, PGCEA, MILT, Head of Department of Health and Social Welfare, Christchurch Canterbury University College, Kent.

Charlotte Maddison MSc, BA (Hons), RGN, Senior Lecturer, School of Health and Social Care, Oxford Brookes University.

Hazel Platzer RGN, RMN, BA (Hons), MSc, PGCE (A), Independent Research Consultant and Trainer.

Pam Sharp MSc, PG Dip, RGN, Senior Lecturer, School of Health and Social Care. Oxford Brookes University.

Sue Schutz MSc, RGN, Cert Ed (FE), Senior Lecturer, School of Health and Social Care, Oxford Brookes University.

Preface

'... A process of reviewing an experience of practice in order to describe, analyse and evaluate and so inform learning from practice'

(Reid 1993, p.305)

Welcome to the third edition of *Reflective Practice in Nursing*. In keeping with the definition of reflection-on-action quoted above, this is a book about learning from experience. This new edition responds to the interest among nurses to master the fundamental skills of reflective practice. It offers a motivating and accessible text that documents and analyses the increase in knowledge and skills surrounding reflection, which has been developing since the early 1990s. We hope it continues to provide a route to communicate our growing knowledge and expertise about reflective practice which originated in nurse education at Oxford Brookes University and its collaborating NHS Trusts, both of which value and support the development of reflective practice. Fundamentally this book does not assume any previous knowledge about reflection and aims to provide a text of practical use to those wanting to learn about reflection and what it may have to offer them.

Past editions of *Reflective Practice in Nursing* have been read by a wide variety of nurses: pre and post-registration students, and from diploma to master's level. The book has had appeal for practitioners from a huge range of backgrounds and experience, as well as for teachers, managers and mentors and professionals from other disciplines. The success of the previous editions has motivated us to continue to communicate our experience, and growing expertise and knowledge in using reflective practice. Although more research in the area is still needed (indeed this is something on our agenda now) our own continuing work and experience with reflective practice keeps us committed to a process that has the potential to help nurses to learn from their practice.

We hope this third edition has much to offer. We have concentrated on updating readers with much of the latest nursing research on reflection, as well as offering some fundamental information and critical analysis on its theoretical underpinnings (Chapter 1). This is useful if you are new to reflection and also for re-examining your thinking if you have some experience of it already. The chapter on skills for reflection (Chapter 2) has been updated; along with help to develop your self-awareness, description, critical analysis, synthesis and evaluation skills, there are some extra pointers on how you can influence change as a reflective practitioner. The challenging chapter on assessing and evaluating reflection (Chapter 3) remains and has been added to and updated. This is a difficult area for debate but we feel it needs to continue to be raised, if practice knowledge is to be valued in the same way as theoretical knowledge. We have also amalgamated work on mentors and supervision into one chapter concerned with supporting practitioners in the process of reflection (Chapter 4); this work draws on the author's research as well as her experience and critique of the literature. In response to readers' comments we have added new chapters on writing for reflection (Chapter 5) and on group reflection (Chapter 6); these offer plenty of advice and tips for practitioners and educationalists, as well as a lively critique.

We continue to present an evaluative look at the experiences of students involved in developing their practice; however in this edition we have concentrated on pre-registration undergraduates and for the first time have included the experiences of teachers involved in reflective education (Chapter 7). This ongoing work presents a fascinating insight into the reality of reflection for those involved in teaching and learning about it. Again, we think there is much inspiration to be gained from the chapter continuing to explore our intrepid practitioner's reflections as she progresses with her career (Chapter 8). Sue Duke offers some useful insights into her practice and some strategies for focusing and progressing with one's reflection.

Finally, there is a chapter which gives some condensed guidance (Chapter 9), drawing on other areas of the book and giving plenty of hints, tips and cautions for getting started with some reflections of your own. This chapter includes new and old exemplars to continue to give an insight into other people's reflection and to provide a resource for teachers and students. Our thanks to Kerry Davidson, Paul Emmanuel, Debbie Holm, Rachel King and Gerry Linke, who have all contributed their reflective writing to share with others.

Reflection is not without its critics; indeed we hope that we have managed to convey the problematic issues, as well as the positive aspects. Healthy debate and critical discussion are important and we hope you get a sense of this as you compare and contrast the views of different contributors to this book. In essence, our aim is to make you curious about reflection in a way that gets you thinking about the issues involved and challenges you to look at your view of the world. Essentially, we hope it will be useful to all those involved and interested in developing, using and investigating reflective practice.

Reference

Reid B (1993) 'But we're doing it already!' Exploring a response to the concept of reflective practice in order to improve its facilitation. *Nurse Education Today*, 13, 305–9.

Chapter 1
An Introduction to Reflection

Chris Bulman

Introduction

Reflection is undoubtedly an important concept in nursing and since the first edition of this book, published in 1994, reflection has succeeded in stimulating debate and investigation, and influencing nursing education around the world. It has got 'under the skin' of practitioners and educationalists in an amazing way considering the amount of critical debate it has aroused and the lack of empirical work investigating the concept through research. It is a concept that we remain committed to, hence the development of this book documenting our experiences, exploring the theoretical debates, reviewing the latest research and offering advice and discussion on reflection and reflective education.

We hope this book will help you to make up your own mind about reflection, because we have critiqued some of the issues, put forward some theoretical background in order to help you get a grasp of what reflection is and encouraged you to have a go at it. It is, as always, wise to use your own informed judgement to work out what you think about reflection, otherwise as FitzGerald and Chapman (2000) caution, one prevalent discourse simply replaces another and the ideas associated with that dominant discourse become so influential that alternative views, especially minority views, are in danger of being marginalised. Words of caution aside, in producing this book we are in effect 'declaring our hand' in that we obviously believe there are benefits to be gained from using reflection; however we are aware of the difficulties as well, which any good academic and practical debate should not ignore.

Current thinking in nursing advocates the need for nurses to be educated in ways that develop their autonomy, critical thinking, sensitivity to others and their open-mindedness (Reed & Ground 1997). Reflective education could certainly be a way of achieving this. Consequently, nurses along with other professionals have been interested in and have contributed to the growing body of literature on reflection (e.g. Burns & Bulman 2000; Ghaye & Lilyman 2000; Johns 2000; Bolton 2001; Rolfe *et al.* 2001) because potentially it provides them with a vehicle through which they can communicate and justify the importance of practice and practice knowledge, thus legitimising the knowledge that derives from the realities of practice rather than purely from more traditional forms of knowing. Nursing education has subsequently begun to integrate reflection-on-action (or experience) into the preparation and continuing professional development of nurses (UKCC 1994, 1996).

What is reflection?

Getting to grips with the concept of reflection is a useful starting point, so long as you bear in mind Chris Johns' (2000, p.34) warning against accepting definitions at face value and his comment that practitioners may grasp at theoretical defini- tions and then struggle to fit the experiences to the definition, rather than using the definition to creatively guide reflection. In fact reflection is a difficult concept to define (James & Clarke 1994; Clarke *et al.* 1996) and consequently it is interpreted in the literature in slightly different ways.

The educationalist and philosopher John Dewey developed his ideas on think- ing and learning and focused on the concept of thinking reflectively, defining it as:

'Active, persistent and careful consideration of any belief or supposed form of knowledge in the light of the grounds that support it and the further conclusions to which it tends.'

(Dewey 1933, p.9)

He saw reflective thinking as thinking with a purpose and focused strongly on the need to test out and challenge true beliefs by applying the scientific method through deductive reasoning and experimentation. He implied that emotions and feelings are part of reflective thinking but, interestingly, this is not something on which he expanded. He made some important assumptions about people, emphasising our tendencies towards quick solutions, tradition and 'mental ruts' and the pervading influence of culture and the environment upon our thinking. He also emphasised the need for thinking to be directly linked with action, demon- strating the pragmatic nature of his philosophy, and suggested that any thinking can be intellectual, thus emphasising the importance of the practical as well as the theoretical. His philosophy has had a major influence on educational ideas and certainly influenced the work of Donald Schön (1983, 1987), Boyd and Fales (1983) and Boud *et al.* (1985).

Schön defines *reflection-on-action* as:

'thinking back on what we have done in order to discover how our knowing in action may have contributed to an unexpected outcome. We may do so after the fact, in tranquillity or we may pause in the midst of action (stop and think).'

(Schön 1987, p.26)

His concept of reflection-on-action focuses on retrospective critical thinking, to construct and reconstruct events in order to develop oneself as a practitioner and person. Importantly reflection-on-action involves more than 'intellectual' thinking because it is intermingled with the practitioner's feelings and emotions and acknowledges an inter-relationship with action (Dewey 1933, Schön 1983, 1987).

Schön also defines *reflection-in-action* as happening:

'where we may reflect in the midst of action without interrupting it. Our thinking serves to reshape what we are doing while we are doing it.'

(Schön 1987, p.26)

This is a different concept, as you can see, from reflection-on-action since it is not about carrying out a 'post mortem' (however speedy) on an experience, but concerns thinking and knowing in the midst of action. Schön saw reflection-in-action as a distinguishing feature of expert practitioners who are able to experiment and think about their practice while they are doing it; this idea is fundamental to his theory of professional expertise. This is difficult to conceptualise and you will find it is sometimes misrepresented by those who view reflection-on-action and reflection-in-action as the same, and there are authors who critique the whole concept of reflection-in-action (Eraut 1994; Clinton 1998). In this book our main concerns are with the construction of rational and affective knowledge in order to make a positive difference to practice, and thus you will find that authors within these pages are mainly talking about reflection-on-action.

Nurses have also attempted to offer a definition of reflection based on their interpretation of the theorists and on their own experiences. While working as a practitioner, Brigid Reid formulated a definition after reviewing the work of Boyd and Fales (1983) and Boud *et al.* (1985), in order to develop a working definition that captured theoretical interpretation and could also be used to teach and facilitate nurses learning about reflection for the first time:

> 'Reflection is a process of reviewing an experience of practice in order to describe, analyse, evaluate and so inform learning about practice.'
>
> (Reid 1993, p.306)

The definitions of reflection given by the educationalists that she used are:

> 'Reflective learning is the process of internally examining and exploring an issue of concern, triggered by an experience, which creates and clarifies meaning in terms of self and which results in a changed conceptual perspective.'
>
> (Boyd and Fales 1983, p.113)

> 'Reflection in the context of learning is a generic term for those intellectual and affective activities in which individuals engage to explore their experiences in order to lead to new understandings and appreciations.'
>
> Boud *et al.* (1985, p.19)

Saylor (1990, p.8) is another nurse who attempts a definition of reflection. She was influenced by the work of Donald Schön and draws on her own experience as a nurse teacher:

> 'Reflection is a process of reviewing one's repertoire of clinical experience and knowledge to invent novel approaches to complex clinical problems. Reflection also provides data for self-evaluation and increases learning from experience.'

Additionally Clarke and Graham (1996, p.26) define the process of reflection:

> 'By engaging in reflection people are usually engaging in a period of thinking in order to examine often complex experiences or situations. The period of thinking (reflection) allows the individual to make sense of an experience, perhaps to liken the experience to other similar experiences and to place it in context. Faced with complex decisions thinking it through (reflecting) allows

the individual to separate out the various influencing factors and come to a reasoned decision or course of action.'

Wong *et al.* (1997) describe the central point of reflection as experience, with the trigger point of the process usually starting with an emotional response (Dewey 1933), which can be both positive (Boud *et al.* 1985) and uncomfortable (Atkins & Murphy 1993). Like Clarke and Graham they describe the reflective process as one of making sense of an experience and learning from it.

There are others you will come across in the literature; however if you were expecting to find one universal definition of reflection you will be disappointed. Some things are hard to define and so a unanimously agreed definition for reflection may not be a possibility. Maybe we would do well to pay more attention to how we as nurses identify the meaning of reflection within our practice and what similarities and differences we recognise in our interpretations, (Wittgenstein 1967). If you look carefully at the definitions presented above, you will begin to notice some similarities; for instance, the exploration of experience, the analysis of feelings or of self to inform learning. You will also see elements of critical theory where there is an assumption that reflection will involve a changed perspective and action. It is also possible to see elements of experimentation and review and learning through one's experience. There are inevitably differences in the definitions too: for instance, not all emphasise the importance of feelings and emotion, or overtly recognise the inclusion of change. So it seems to me that it is necessary to do some reading for yourself, as well as taking a look at how you personally operate in practice, to begin to consider what you make of reflection.

In simple terms, I see reflection-on-action as reviewing experience from practice so that it may be described, analysed, evaluated and consequently used to inform and change future practice. It also involves opening up our practice for others to examine and consequently requires courage and open-mindedness as well as a willingness to take on board and act on criticism (Dewey 1933). Reflection in this context involves more than 'intellectual thinking' but is intermingled with practitioners' feelings and emotions and acknowledges the interrelationship with action. Grasping the idea that reflection is a combination of thinking, emotion and commitment to action is not an easy one and a look at the philosophical legacy around thinking and knowing is helpful.

The philosophical legacy surrounding thinking and knowing and why it is important to reflection

Taking a look at the philosophical ideas surrounding thinking and knowing reveals some interesting issues. Some of this legacy promotes the notion that intellectual knowledge is different from, and indeed is superior to, practical knowledge and denies an interrelationship between intellect and emotion. It can be seen to originate from the work of early western philosophers such as Plato, focusing on the domination of intellectual inquiry in the search for the 'truth' about knowledge (Day 1994), but is strongly influenced by later Cartesian theory which views the mind as separate from the body. Descartes was a rationalist (truth is revealed through reason), scientist and deductive thinker; his belief in God developed his thinking around the human soul or mind being divine and the need to have the mind uncontaminated by the sensual nature of the body. He is famously remembered for his proposition 'I am thinking therefore I am', identifying the soul or mind as something separate from the body. It was Descartes' propositions that promoted the concept of dualism focusing on 'thinking skills' as separate from the body. Ironically, in some of his later work Descartes did begin to explore the union between mind and body; however, philosophers could be accused of ignoring this aspect of Descartes' work and focusing instead on his propositions surrounding dualism (Cottingham 1997).

The influence of dualism pervades many aspects of life today and perhaps would be best recognised among nurses in the development of the mind–body split in early conceptions of medicine; some may even say that the dualistic viewpoint still exists today with the split being made between the brain and the body rather than the mind and body! The enduring nature of Descartes' propositions may have much to do with the influence of religion and the need to justify the notion of the immortal soul as well as the dominance of intellectual knowledge over the practical and emotional.

Later philosophers began to appreciate thinking from an inherently different stance, arguing that the mind and body are interconnected and that knowledge is socially rather than individually constructed and thus thinking, emotion and action are intertwined (Ryle 1963; Wittgenstein 1967). Wittgenstein for instance identified that it is people and not minds that think, feel and act and that human behaviour is bound up with thinking, emotion and meaning. He suggested that we use imagination, judgement and self-reflection to make sense of the world. His ideas are important because they provide a route for describing thinking and knowing that takes into account its social context, emphasising the need to describe people, their behaviour and their language in order to understand meaning.

Gilbert Ryle famously disagreed with the Cartesian approach to philosophy, dismissing the theological concept of the human soul and criticising the concepts of the mind, consciousness and the subjective experience. His phrase the 'ghost in the machine' encapsulates his critique of Descartes, challenging the notion of the mind or 'ghost' that owns or controls the body (Ryle 1963). In arguing against the ideals of dualism, where mental performance is separate from the physical, he suggested that intelligent action or thinking can be seen in people's behaviour, so that people can demonstrate their knowledge through their capacities, skills and habits, thus interlinking mind and body. Ryle also advocated the need to look at imagination or improvisation and critical thinking as elements of, not as different types of, thinking.

My very brief look at some philosophical influences is included to highlight the argument that reflection cannot just be about our cognitive ability. If you follow the argument presented above, it has to include affective elements as well as an acknowledgement of action. Reflective thinking highlights the intermingling of practitioners' feelings and emotions, and acknowledges this interrelationship with action as well as the importance of intellectual thinking. It provides a vehicle for legitimising professional knowledge that develops from the realities of practice and challenges more traditional forms of knowing.

Nursing, higher education and a challenge to traditional views of critical thinking

The legacy of Cartesian theory is powerful despite developments in post-modern philosophy. The superiority of intellectual knowledge in education therefore remains strong (Brockbank & McGill 1998). Consequently nursing education exists within a higher education system that historically promotes the division between theoretical and practical knowledge and which traditionally denies a relationship between intellect and emotion. Reflective education, however, potentially provides a way to justify the importance of practice and recognises the interrelationship between theoretical and practical knowledge, embracing the intermingling of thinking, emotion and action. Thus, reflective practice provides a justification for practice knowledge and is appealing to us as nurses because we are able to identify with this.

Nursing, of course, is a practice discipline and effective preparation of nurses requires that we are able to care competently for our clients and continue to develop our skills and knowledge over a professional lifetime. This means that we need to learn certain skills and particular knowledge, and develop attitudes and attributes that allow us to nurse in an effective and sensitive way that makes a difference to our clients (Paterson and Zderad 1988; McMahon & Pearson 1998). A traditional way of achieving this is through what Schön (1983, 1987) would call technical rationality, where students learn about theory and then apply this to their practice, echoing the stance of dualism and the separation of intellectual and practical knowledge as outlined above. Many of you who have experienced traditional nursing courses will be able to identify with this style of education.

In higher education there has been a change of climate generally, challenging the traditional notion of 'banking' education as defined by Friere (1972) where students are filled up with knowledge and teachers are the givers of such knowledge. There is more emphasis on and interest in enabling students to develop skills that help them 'learn how to learn', through developing good critical thinking (Barnett 1992). Additionally, there is educational research and theory that advocates the importance and effectiveness of learning through experience (Jarvis 1983; Rogers 1983; Gibbs 1988). So it is difficult from this perspective to believe that thinking critically about practice in order to learn and develop from it, is a misplaced concept in the education of professionals. Indeed, if it is possible to appreciate the flaws presented by dualism where thinking is seen only as intellectual and is separated from emotion and action, then logically it is also possible to imply that critical thinking can never be fully rational, linear and grounded totally in a scientific approach. This leads neatly towards a brief but critical consideration of the work of Donald Schön, an influential figure in the development of present ideas on reflective practice in nursing. His work is much quoted in the literature and has been an inspiration to the development of reflective practice in nursing and other professions. So it is valuable to present his ideas because they offer some useful insights into the utility and popularity of reflection.

A brief look at Schön

Schön believed that practice should be central to professional curricula, a point that presumably most professionals would agree with. Consequently he saw learning by doing becoming the core of programmes rather than an add-on, with students investing in practice and putting in time in order to learn from it. This offers a slightly different focus from reliance on a competency based curriculum since it implies that students need to develop a commitment to practice and the motivation to learn from it. As you will see, Schön's work focused on the use of practica in education and not on the real world of practice. Additionally Schön saw the artistry of coaching as really important to the development of students' learning.

Professional knowledge

Schön's work suggested a crisis in confidence in professional knowledge, and he commented that:

> 'When professionals fail to recognise and respond to value conflicts, when they violate their own ethical standards, fall short of self-directed expectations for expert performance; or seem blind to public problems they have helped to create, they are increasingly subject to expressions of disapproval and dissatisfaction.'

(Schön 1987, p.7)

He raised Ivan Illich's criticism of professionals as misappropriating and monopolising knowledge, disregarding social injustices and mystifying expertise; but he also pointed out the tensions for professions, such as facing increasing expectations from the public and working in large bureaucratic organisations. He suggested that these conflicts and tensions call for a radical rethink in the manner in which we develop and understand the ways that professionals practise.

He also believed that what aspiring professionals need most, professional schools seem least able to teach and he attributed this to an underlying, largely unexamined, epistemology of professional practice. He suggested that professional curricula and arrangements for research and practice are premised on the concept of technical rationality where practical competence can be seen to be achieved through instrumental problem solving grounded in systematic, preferably scientific knowledge. Schön (1983, 1987), saw this as a flawed view of professional competence and its relationship to scientific and scholarly research.

Professional artistry

So he coined the phrase 'professional artistry', firstly that we can recognise artistry in certain unusually competent individuals; and secondly that artistry is a kind of knowing but is different from the standard model of professional knowledge. In order to learn more about artistry, he suggested studying the performance of unusually competent performers. He believed that there is an art to problem framing, implementation and improvisation and that these are all necessary in order to use applied science and technique in practice.

Schön suggested that professional artistry can be understood in terms of reflection-in-action. He saw reflection-in-action as constructionist where the professional constructs situations from practice as opposed to technical rationality which rests on an objectivist view (facts are what they are and the truth of beliefs is strictly testable by reference to them). He believed that professionals construct their reality of practice via their perceptions, appreciations and beliefs rooted in their own world and this is what they come to accept as their own reality.

What did Schön mean by a practicum?

Schön suggested that professional education should be able to teach students about the artistry of practice and he advocated practicum-based coaching as a means of doing so (a practicum is a setting designed for the task of learning practice). In the practicum, students learn from those with more experience in practice; his examples are practica where coaching can be carried out in a relatively low risk environment, for example an artist's studio, design studio or classroom supervision session. He turned his attention to coaching in architecture, musical performance, psychoanalytic supervision and group work and his own seminar work with Chris Argyris, in an attempt to make a case for his theoretical arguments. His work emphasises the importance of the coaching element in reflection, where students can be both supported and challenged, thus developing the critical element of reflection. Schön's view of the practicum would equate with nursing education in the skills laboratory, group work using case studies, critically analysing practice, but not with direct practice where students learn about nursing in the real world. Quite rightly he talked about this preparation as having to be more than applying facts, rules and procedures and saw it as an opportunity for students learning to think.

High hard ground and swampy lowlands

Schön described professional practice as a high hard ground overlooking a swamp, where the high ground represents manageable problems that lend themselves to solution through applying research-based technique and theory. The swampy lowland denotes messy confusing problems that defy technical solution. In fact, he suggested that the problems of real world practice do not tend to present themselves as problems at all but as messy indeterminate situations. His powerful metaphor is one with which professionals have been able to identify.

Schön saw professionals naming and framing problems in order to deal with them and noticed that the way this is handled varies between disciplines, in how professionals are prepared and in individual ways of looking at the world. Consequently, practice problems are not dealt with in exactly the same way by all professionals, and professional practice cannot be seen as just the application of technical rationality to practice problems. So he does not discount technical rationality but rather he makes a case for it not being the entire solution for many of the problems in the chaotic complexities of the real world.

Reflection-in-action and reflection-on-action

While Schön acknowledges that reflection-on-action is useful for the development of reflective practitioners, he does not particularly focus on this area of reflection, preferring it seems to concentrate on describing the artistry of practice through the use of reflection-in-action. Schön urged the need for a new epistemology of practice where professional education combines the teaching of applied science with coaching, in the artistry of reflection-in-action, in order to equip professionals with the skills and knowledge to work effectively within the realities of the practice world.

In order to further demonstrate his vision of reflection-in action, he acknowledged the importance of knowing-in-action, suggesting that when you see a skilled performance, the knowing is in the action (presumably influenced by the work of people like Gilbert Ryle); however, it is characteristically difficult to make this verbally explicit. Eraut (1994) points out this issue, suggesting that once we begin to think about our thinking and attempt to communicate this through the reflective process, the nature of knowledge changes from tacit (Polanyi 1967) and spontaneous to explicit and symbolic. This is because, as Schön suggests, it has moved from knowing-in-action, to speaking or writing about knowing-in-action. Thus Schön makes the important point that once knowing is communicated to the social world its very nature is altered. This is complicated by the fact that we do not always know what we know and this consequently raises problems when it comes to communicating this to others or making sense of it through our own thinking, a paradox first raised by Plato and picked up by Schön through his work.

Schön acknowledged the difficulties of giving a good verbal description of something and comments on skilful improvisers often becoming tongue-tied or giving obviously inadequate accounts when asked to say what they do. This emphasises the difficulties of trying to get to grips with Schön's concept of reflection-in-action and relates back to the fact that we do not sometimes know what we know, and that once knowledge is in the social domain it is no longer tacit.

Some issues with Schön

Schön's philosophical arguments are of real interest to professionals and no doubt many would identify with the premises he makes about the nature of professional practice. However, the theoretical strength of his work is not reflected in the examples he gives describing reflective practice and the education of professionals. His examples of coaching are not well described and they do not appear to be particularly facilitative. I believe that there is some confusion in Schön's attempts to describe coaching, confusing this with the performance of the skilful practitioner; the two are not the same.

Presumably Schön is working from the premise that knowing can be seen through purposeful action, as described by Ryle, but even Ryle (1979) acknowledges the limits of purely describing what can be seen. This is because of such issues as negative action, where people make an active decision not to do something and this cannot be seen in their behaviour, and also the need to look beyond the performance itself and be aware of people's abilities and predispositions. Additionally, in the real world of practice one cannot easily experiment rigorously, especially where the welfare of people is concerned. Schön does suggest however that the practitioner draws on his or her repertoire of experience as well as the theory that he or she is committed to and feels relevant to his or her practice, again a proposition that practitioners could identify with.

Eraut (1994) is more critical of Schön's work, believing that he moves away from his own definitions and evidence, making statements that are difficult to defend. Eraut suggests that Schön offers no coherent view of reflection but instead gives a set of overlapping attributes, selecting those attributes that best suit his situation under discussion. Eraut suggests that even Schön himself does not always differentiate between 'in' and 'on' action and that his only consistency is in the 'reframing of a problem'. Eraut suggests taking the term reflection out of Schön's theory and instead thinking of his work as a theory of metacognition or thinking about thinking, but this viewpoint fails to capture the emotional and action element associated with reflection. He goes on to suggest that Schön's reflection-on-action is less problematic, where one makes sense of an action after it has occurred, learning something from it and extending one's knowledge base. However, he does ask what Schön actually means by action, since action could mean anything from one incident to several months of accumulating experience or a whole lifetime of practice. In fact, it is my experience that people are able to reflect across this whole range from one incident to their practice in general.

Eraut suggests that Schön ignores the time element of quick decision-making, something which Eraut sees as a fundamental part of many professionals' working realities. He criticises Schön's assumption that the process is analytical and critical and this is certainly an issue picked up in subsequent nursing research, as you will see below. He also points out that many of the coaching examples presented by Schön do not echo the practice situations of many professionals. This is true in some ways as we have taken a leap of faith in using these ideas in the nursing practice setting where there are pros and cons, as you will see in later chapters; however, they are still used a great deal within group work, classroom discussion and skills laboratory work. He also suggests that Schön makes the mistake of transferring expertise in clinical practice into expertise in coaching students without supporting evidence and sometimes in the face of indications to the contrary; this raises the very important point that not all experts necessarily make good coaches.

Further reading of Schön for yourself will of course help you to make up your own mind on the implications of his work. His ideas have certainly been an inspiration to many, including ourselves, but it is important to bear in mind both their strengths and weaknesses.

Stages and levels of reflection

Various authors have published work on stages and levels of reflection and these theoretical approaches have been taken up by researchers and educationalists in their attempts to capture the development of reflective ability (Van Manen 1977; Mesirow 1981; Goodman 1984; James & Clarke 1994; Kim 1999). They do, however, make the reductionist assumption that reflection can be regarded in terms of stages and levels. You will find these authors mentioned throughout the book, and more detail and discussion on Goodman's and Mesirow's work is given in Chapter 9 since they offer useful frameworks for qualifying reflection.

Skills necessary for reflection

A review of the literature by Atkins and Murphy (1993) enabled them to make some suggestions about the sorts of skills that might be fundamental to developing reflective practice. These are self-awareness, description, critical analysis, synthesis, judgement and evaluation. Elements of these skills are discussed in many of the nursing research studies to date but again more work would be welcome in this area. Chapter 2 in this book provides much more detail about Sue Atkins' ideas surrounding the skills necessary for reflection.

Nursing research

The body of nursing research in reflection is growing, however it still needs to be viewed tentatively since a number of the papers lack quality in their design or in some cases the research is so briefly described that it is difficult to judge its quality (a problem with publications rather than the study perhaps?). The research is mainly qualitative, reflecting the need to explore an area in nursing where little previous work has been carried out. There is more research evidence on the use of clinical supervision using a reflective approach, and the work of Johns (1993, 1994, 1995a,b, 2000; Johns & Freshwater 1998) would be a good place to start if you wish to explore this area of nursing research.

Much of the research reviewed here is small scale with the majority of researchers recognising the lack of generalisability in their work. Many of the studies are carried out by educationalists who are often researching their own students and thus there may be issues of bias. One of the most noticeable factors with many of the studies is the lack of information given on their research design, particularly how researchers analysed their data and how they extrapolated their findings from their analysis. The other evident factor is that researchers on the whole do not offer a great deal of detail or evidence about how nurses were actually prepared and facilitated to develop reflection. With all good intention, they tend to focus on outcome, thus there is less nursing research evidence about the process of reflection.

Criticisms aside, Heath (1998) describes the nursing literature generally as urging the need for research that demonstrates large and rapid benefits with measurable outcomes, and that small accumulated gains are not considered good enough. However, the reality of knowledge development is often that evidence is built up by slow accumulation over time, so the promise of one big wonderful study that demonstrates that reflection makes a difference to client care once and for all, is not a realistic option. Heath suggests that there is repeated concern for reflection to demonstrate positive outcomes in client care; however, she also suggests that the processes of care and outcome are complex and that the effect of reflection in terms of precise measurement and separation from other factors is difficult to achieve (see Chapter 3 for more detail on this). Therefore she recommends the need to focus on the development of practitioners accepting the assumption that enhancing skills will lead to better patient care.

Nursing research involving reflective diaries or journals

The use of reflective journals or diaries has been explored with varying findings. Generally students appear to find the use of reflective journals helpful; however, it is unclear whether diaries and journals support the development of deeper levels of critical thinking and there are issues surrounding the assessment of what constitute private diaries (McCaugherty 1991; Landeen *et al.* 1995; Richardson & Maltby 1995; Shields 1995; Clarke & Graham 1996; Durgahee 1996; Riley-Doucet & Wilson 1997; Wong *et al.* 1997; Fonteyn & Cahill 1998). See Chapters 3 and 5 for more debate about this.

One of the more rigorous studies is that of Wong *et al.* (1997) who found in their action research study in Hong Kong that journals written by nurses were very descriptive to begin with and students failed to integrate literature with their practical experience. Students were then asked to focus on critical incidents related to a particular theme and to take part in group discussions related to them; this new strategy was found helpful. As time went on, differences in reflective ability among students, based on the work of Mesirow (1981), began to emerge, 70% were identified as reflectors, with one seventh of these particularly identified as critical reflectors, and approximately 30% of students were identified at the lower levels of reflective learning. Reflectors had two main attributes, willingness and commitment to endeavour and open-mindedness. Richardson and Maltby (1995) found a similar spread of reflective ability in students' diary reflections. Again they used the work of Mesirow as adapted by Powell (1989), and found that most students (94%) only demonstrated lower levels of reflection, with only 6% found to demonstrate the higher levels of reflection involving critical consciousness.

Fonteyn and Cahill (1998), in a North American study, explored the use of clinical logs as an alternative to written care plans to help students develop thinking strategies and metacognitive skills. They found that students preferred the clinical reflective logs and did develop their thinking. However, the students' levels of thinking demonstrated do seem unsophisticated for their level of training and do not reveal any considerations of feelings about practice experiences which would indicate the affective component of reflective thinking. Durgahee (1996) found that diaries helped students to think about their practice and acted as a consciousness raising tool; after a year, diaries showed that students seemed to have acquired a more critical thinking pattern. However, initially diary keeping caused some anxiety and confusion, and students needed to develop their observational and analysis skills. Even after a year, some still had difficulties with their diary and some questioned the value of reflective learning. Although reflection generally appeared to help students question and challenge their practice, lack of time and the distractions of practice were cited as things which encroached on opportunities to reflect.

Clarke and Graham (1996) found that nurses in their study also experienced initial difficulties in reflecting and writing a diary. However, participants found acknowledging and accepting feelings and emotions useful, expressed improvement in their critical ability and felt they had developed new insights, ideas and alternative courses of action. They also found their decision-making was enhanced and that frameworks and guidelines based on Atkins and Murphy (1993), Johns (1993) and Schön (1992) were helpful in guiding their reflection. A study by Shields (1995) reveals that students who kept reflective style journals developed their problem solving, personal development and self-analysis through the process of reflection. Three students found mental previewing helpful; most theory on reflection-on-action concentrates on looking back over an event and reflection-pre-action is largely ignored, a point amply made by Greenwood (1998), albeit from a dualistic viewpoint where thinking is separated from feelings and action.

Nursing research exploring writing reflectively

Several studies look at writing reflectively and there is some evidence that having to write reflectively for assignments is viewed positively by nurses, helping to organise and formulate their ability to express themselves (Jasper 1999; Paget 2001). Jasper's grounded theory study also demonstrates the need for reflective writing skills to be learnt. In her study nurses saw writing as facilitating learning, as a process in its own right, and reflective writing was seen to contribute to the facilitation of personal development. Her research uncovered suggestions that writing may provide a mechanism for the development of analytical and critical skills that impact on nurses' practice, and that reflective writing helped nurses to explore themselves. This was potentially seen as threatening but was an avenue for admitting strengths and weaknesses and developing them as a result. All 16 nurses in this study felt they had changed and developed as people through their reflective writing. This study illustrates Heath's point above about the difficulties of being able to exclude other factors that may develop participants' learning and practice. In this case, participants were taking a one-year research course using reflection, and consequently it is difficult to rule out the effect of their new research knowledge and skills on reported changes.

A well-written quantitative study by Duke and Appleton (2000), examining the development of palliative care students' reflective writing over time, demonstrated that nurses' reflective skills did develop over time but again that skills indicative of critical reflection were less evident and confined to the ability to raise implications for future learning. While students were able to describe their practice, their ability to analyse knowledge and the content of care and action planning was not so well achieved. As the researchers point out, these latter abilities are all crucial skills in the development of critical reflection. The researchers also suggest that students' lack of action planning could be due to their viewing the reflective learning contract as an academic exercise rather than as a way of developing their practice, or it could be that students feel powerless to change things. The researchers point out two important issues that hamper the development of research into reflection, namely making the reductionist assumption that reflection can be divided into skills and that those assessing other's written reflection are able to differentiate consistently between the different skills being assessed.

Spencer and Newell's (1999) quasi-experimental pilot study demonstrated that nurses' reflective writing skills improved following long distance learning packages, and they noted that participants often wrote positive things about themselves and negative things about others. However, the researchers do not consider the coaching and facilitation elements associated with reflection, and approach it more as a technical skill which can be learnt without a relationship between nurse, supervisor or teacher. This is a stance that many of the more humanistic writers on reflection would no doubt take issue with. There are also some issues of self-selection bias and low inter-rater reliability in this quantitative study.

Sorrell *et al.* (1997) adopt a slightly different approach to assessing students' written reflective abilities. Students were asked to submit a portfolio of work that they felt demonstrated their critical thinking, plus a reflective essay. Students viewed critical thinking as 'seeing in a special way', and they were able to identify it as an analytic process but also a creative one. Interestingly, students viewed their more scholarly research papers as most evident of critical thinking. However, educationalists who also evaluated their work saw most evidence of critical thinking in their clinical examples of writing. The most fascinating thing about this study is that this was more clearly seen by the professors of English who took part in the study than by the professors of nursing! Despite these findings, it was evident that most of the assignments remained descriptive in nature. This study does demonstrate some confusion between critical thinking and reflection, with the two at times being used interchangeably; it also shows in particular how easy it is to adopt a dualistic approach to reflection and critical thinking.

Finally, Kember *et al.* (1996) contribute an action research project from Hong Kong, developing curricula to encourage students to write reflective journals. They examined five different health care professional courses including nursing, in an ongoing project. Their findings to date revealed that the development of reflective writing took time and for some was hard to achieve. Unlearning the impersonal style of academic writing was hard for some students, but with careful instructional planning and frequent feedback, students were able to achieve it. As well as space and time to allow the development of reflective writing, students also benefited from frequent feedback from teachers, clinical supervisors and peers. The development of reflective writing was more successful in courses where journal keeping was a central and important feature, and less successful where this was treated as a voluntary exercise, posing an additional burden of work for students. This study offers some useful, articulate and in depth description of the findings, illuminated by narrative examples. However, there is very little information about the research design, particularly concerning issues of ethical rigor, details of decision-making, sampling and the handling of data analysis.

Nursing research exploring group reflection

Studies looking at group reflection appear to indicate the supportive elements of group discussion and analysis, as well as the difficulties of revealing thoughts and feelings and adjusting to a more student centred approach to learning (Snowball *et al.* 1994; Clarke & Graham 1996; Mountford & Rogers 1996; Hayes 1998; Graham 2000; Page & Meerabeau 2000; Platzer *et al.* 2000a,b; Hyrkas *et al.* 2001; Paget 2001).

Clarke and Graham (1996) found that reflective group tutorials were influential in promoting trust, honesty and openness, but that lecturers needed good facilitation skills in order to deal with emotional and difficult issues. Graham (2000) facilitated group reflection over a year in a nursing development unit, using a qualitative approach; very little detail is given on research design for the study but findings suggest that the process was highly successful, giving staff insights into the nature of nursing and their practice. The group meetings helped to develop professional cohesion and identity and staff had the opportunity to articulate theory underpinning their practice; interestingly, nurses did not usually share their experiences of working with patients. The process also focused thinking and highlighted the nurses' awareness of their inability to change certain things, thus echoing a point about powerlessness in Duke and Appleton's study.

Hayes (1998) facilitated a reflective group for forensic psychiatric nurses over a period of two months, while members found the group supportive, reflecting on critical incidents raised powerful negative emotions in group members. There were also indications that group members did not always reach critical levels of reflection, similar to the findings in some of the studies above; however, members were able to see the educational value of reflection. Hayes' discussion focuses on the importance of good facilitation for such groups, and more detail of this from his study would have been valuable. Platzer *et al.* (2000a,b) evaluated group reflection on a post-registration diploma course and also highlight the need for appropriate facilitation of group reflection (Have a look at Chapter 6 in this book to appreciate more of Hazel Platzer's insights into group reflection). Their study suggests that students may have to overcome many barriers to learning before they can benefit from this approach. They refer to previous educational experiences which do not encourage critical thinking or reflection, working cultures that affect people's willingness to expose themselves to judgement and their ability to take responsibility for their own learning. Despite this, reflective groups were a positive experience for most students and the development of critical thinking and perspective transformation did lead to changes in their attitudes and behaviour. Interestingly, some students had begun to change their allegiance from the organisation and their professional groups more towards the interests of their clients, demonstrating the development of a more client centred approach to their attitudes.

Snowball *et al.* (1994) used reflective group work to explore educators' roles as dissertation supervisors; they found that reflection for them was a good tool for learning. They identified a tendency in the group to dwell on the things they were not good at rather than look at their strengths and their need for constructive support. They also identified the need to achieve a balance between self-disclosure and self-enhancement, focusing on the need for a supportive group if the development of self is to be encouraged. Stoddart *et al.* (1996) report some similar issues in their exploration of student nurses' experiences of reflective groups. Students valued the opportunity to talk about problems related to both coursework and practice, but noted the influential nature of the group facilitator in encouraging the group to feel comfortable to open up. Most students found the experience a positive one, but their conceptions of reflection varied and the support they received may have been just because of the group and not necessarily because of the reflective element. While this study has an honest and practical feel to the way it is reported, there is very little information given on its design.

Mountford and Rogers' (1996) study is extensively quoted in the literature, but again contains little information on its design to enable a judgement to be made about quality. In line with other studies, they report that post-registration students found group reflection helpful; students learnt from each other and enjoyed sharing fears, ideas and achievements. These students particularly were characterised as returners to education, experiencing difficulties with gaining knowledge and writing assignments, and reflection was identified as one way of dealing with these issues. Davies *et al.* (1999), in a small action research project, also found that students benefited from reflective teaching sessions shared with mentors and a link lecturer within a gynaecology ward setting. Although the sessions were primarily focused on developing students, mentors also found the chance to think about and review their practice helpful. Mentors also felt the sessions impacted positively on the students' practice and helped them as practitioners to see the students' presence in practice as a positive asset. Francis *et al.* (1998) offer some similar themes found in the other studies above, in their examination of students' philosophies about nursing before and after they had experienced the development of reflective skills through groups and journal writing. Those with little prior experience of adult centred learning had difficulty in constructing reflection as the researchers had defined it, although the majority of students felt that they used reflection naturally. Those that showed a significant change in their philosophies talked about taking time out to reflect and looked at broader aspects rather than immediate issues, describing reflection as a growth process. Again, this study raises some of the difficulties of group work; exposing self was seen as risky – some participants opened up over time, but some did not speak. Development of trust varied between students and this was influenced by the time available and by the facilitator. Knowing self did not necessarily equate with being able to think critically. The important bias of judging participants' values about reflection against the values of the researcher, is noted by the researchers and demonstrates the crucial importance of reflexivity in any qualitative work in this area.

Nursing research exploring reflective education or preparation

Other studies also indicate that reflective learning is a positive and useful experience for students (McCaugherty 1991; Green & Holloway 1997; Hallett 1997; Francis *et al.* 1998, Smith 1998; Davies *et al.* 1999; Glaze 2001a,b; Hart *et al.* 2000; Liimatainen *et al.* 2001, Paget 2001; Suhre & Harskamp 2001). There are also indications that reflective ability takes time to develop but students do report positive changes in their practice as they progress through a reflective education programme (Durgahee 1996; Wong *et al.* 1997; Duke & Appleton 2000; Liimatainen *et al.* 2001; Paget 2001).

Paget's (2001) longitudinal, combined-method study of reflective education found that respondents felt it was the facilitation of reflective education that was a major influence on the outcomes of reflective practice, a point echoed in the findings from group reflection above. Respondents in the study felt that reflective practice did influence their clinical practice, helping them to learn how to learn. They described personal, broad and long-term changes and they continued to change after formal reflection and supervision had finished. Although reflection encouraged respondents to try and change their practice, they were not always successful in this. This perhaps links to studies above that indicate the powerlessness that nurses can feel to change things. A well-written qualitative study by Glaze (2001a,b) also reports MSc Advanced Nursing students' positive experiences of a reflective education. Students described developing greater awareness and appreciation of what nursing could be, becoming more realistic, open and confident, more assertive and enlightened, pushing the boundaries of practice and mentioning the desire to empower staff. Students also described the deepening of their reflection using theory and literature to affirm and explore their ideas. Students used Goodman's (1984) levels of reflection as a framework and this helped to encourage double-loop learning (Argyris & Schön 1974) or critical reflection. One student found the experience difficult; she worked in an oppressive environment and reflection compounded her sense of helplessness, difficulties with writing and her self-assessed negative approach to life. This particular finding serves to highlight the importance of people's environment in encouraging a reflective approach to practice, a point made by several theorists as far back as Dewey (1933). Students also found that reflection was a transformational process, which was demanding and influenced by their personal background. For instance, negative factors inhibiting their reflection were lack of insight, their early nursing socialisation of obedience, prior educational experiences and time. As students responded to challenges in their reflective learning contracts they began to see the ideological factors that constructed their practice and they learnt to reframe their perceptions and were able to describe changes in their thinking and learning.

Hallett (1997) explored P2000 students working with District Nurses as part of a larger ENB study; as students gained experience they began to see links between theory and practice, assisted by their supervisors who encouraged reflection, discussion and questioning and acted as role models. The researcher compares her findings to Schön's theories on reflection and coaching but acknowledges interpretation bias involved in this. While this study does lack design detail, there is some useful narrative included which enhances the presentation of results. Liimatainen *et al.* (2001) use a mixture of observation and interview in their research methods and focus on the development of reflective learning in students within the context of health promotion. Like other researchers, they used the work of Mesirow to assess reflective ability and found that half of the students in the study developed the critical consciousness defined by Mesirow; however, there was evidence of the development of thinking skills in all students. There are some design limitations with this study around lack of follow up of students who dropped out of the study, and the difficulty of pinpointing what exactly made a difference to students' reflective development; however, the longitudinal nature of this study is a positive feature since it is possible to track students' development over time.

Research exploring practising nurses using reflection

A few studies focus on practising nurses who are not engaged in formal education courses (Wallace 1996; Spencer & Newell 1999; Graham 2000; Page & Meerabeau 2000; Teekman 2000), highlighting variations in levels of critical thinking ability as well as both the positive and negative issues involved in reflection around dealing with feelings, the need for support, ability to change practice and integrating theory and practice. A couple of these studies have already been mentioned above. Page and Meerabeau's study explores the use of group reflection with nurses on a cardiac ward. While there was some evidence of improved practice following reflection, it was also evident that required action in practice identified by the group was not always acted upon efficiently; the reticence of the ward leader towards change was also noted. There was a need for trust in the facilitator to allow honest reflection in the group, and sessions were seen to be more for support than for learning. Wallace (1996) reports on her study in progress, with ethnographic data to date demonstrating the importance of recognising and managing feelings in effective reflection, and showing that critical thinking seemed to occur when participants deviated from their expected nursing role, promoting a change in thinking and enhanced care. There is again a lack of detail on design given in this paper and the researcher is working on the assumption that all nurses reflect on their practice.

Teekman (2000) in his qualitative study also explored reflective thinking in nursing practice assuming that it exists without preparation. He did not find critical reflection in his sample of 10 nurses, but only reflection related to action in order move on or keep going in clinical situations; and reflective thinking for evaluation focusing on creating understanding of self and the wholeness of a situation. There is a lack of detail on data analysis in this study and some issues around sample selection; there is also an assumption by the researcher in his discussion that reflection is only a discourse with self, and the coaching and supervision elements of reflection are not considered. Powell (1989) also explores reflection in nurses without any specific preparation and this is the only study that focuses on reflection-in-action in line with Schön's concept of professional artistry. Her findings reveal that reflection-in-action was mainly present in the form of description and in planning actions. Again this qualitative study lacks detail on data analysis, and assumptions are made that appear not to be related to the study findings. This is one of very few studies, however, that tries to combine interviewing and observation to explore nurses' reflection, but this is hampered by issues of bias associated with these methods.

Research exploring nurse teachers

There are very few nursing studies that focus on the experiences and opinions of nurse teachers or how teachers specifically teach reflection-on-action to nurses. More work is needed in this area to explore the need for teachers to be reflective, and to capture their experience of using reflection, their interpretation of reflective theory as well as their ability to teach and facilitate the use of reflection. Burnard (1995) has explored nurse teachers' perceptions of reflection; although the majority of participants were positive and enthusiastic about reflection and teaching reflective practice, there were negative concerns surrounding its unproven value, exposing feelings and intimate values, time, difficulties of recollection and introspection. Participants were also vague about how reflection was actually taught to students and how it could improve clinical practice. While the study has clearly presented themes and narrative which enhance the presentation of the findings, there are indications that the researcher could have probed further to allow participants to elaborate on their responses. This study was conducted some time ago, at a time when reflection was a new concept in nurse education and was beginning to be introduced in nurse teaching; it would be valuable to replicate a similar study today to examine how experiences and opinions have moved on.

Both Scanlan *et al.* (2002) and Snowball *et al.* (1994) explore teachers using reflection. Snowball *et al.*'s (1994) study focuses on the role of reflection for dissertation supervision; reflection proved to be a useful learning tool for the supervisors involved but difficulties were identified, such as the tendency to dwell on the negative rather than look at their strengths as supervisors, as well as the need for constructive support to develop individuals. Findings are clearly presented and well expressed but there is no detail on how supervisors prepared themselves for using reflection or if they shared a common understanding of reflection.

Scanlan *et al.*'s (2002) study focused on the meaning and use of reflection in teaching and how it contributed to the development of teaching expertise in the classroom. Their findings suggested that the more experienced teachers were able to promote and facilitate links between theory and practice more effectively, and that personal reflective abilities did not necessarily transfer to the classroom. Class size and the emotions of the teacher were also found to affect reflection. However, this study does have some limitations; importantly reflection is not explicitly defined as used in the study and so it is difficult to interpret entirely what researchers mean by reflection in the classroom; also, data analysis information is not detailed and consequently it is difficult to appreciate the link between analysis and interpretation.

Hyrkas *et al.* (2001) explored trainee nurse teachers' experiences of reflective teaching and learning in the clinical setting; trainees acted as clinical supervisors to groups of practitioners in ward settings. Trainees felt that the experience enhanced their abilities to work as teachers using reflective strategies with students, and changed their viewpoints about reflection. There is lack of detail on the research design in this study but an honest review of the literature in the paper highlights the need to research the preparation and experience of teachers expected to deliver a reflective curriculum.

Summary of the nursing research findings

A brief look at nursing research within the confines of this chapter reveals the preliminary nature of the body of evidence surrounding reflective practice in nursing. It has begun to demonstrate the pros and cons of a reflective education and we are beginning to learn a little more about its appropriateness and acceptability to students and facilitators. It is an area that needs to be tackled with an appropriate philosophical approach, and does not necessarily attract large amounts of research funding; that said there is certainly room for more.

Conclusion

I hope this introductory chapter gives you an idea of what reflection is, as well as some important underlying theory which will allow you to consider it with a critical eye. It seemed timely to review some of the nursing research in the area, warts and all, so that you can see for yourself where we are in our understanding of reflection in nursing and how nurses have used and interpreted reflective theory. Reflection on experience can, I believe, promote an education where nurses can get to grips with the meaning of their experiences, as well as provide a route whereby we can begin to value our practical expertise as a profession. This requires attention to good facilitation, handy guidance and support in practice and commitment, as well as critique from everyone involved.

References

Argyris, C. & Schön, D. (1974) *Theory in Practice.* Jossey Bass, San Francisco.

Atkins, S. & Murphy, C. (1993) Reflection: a review of the literature. *Journal of Advanced Nursing,* **18** (8), 1188–92.

Barnett, R. (1992) *Improving Higher Education.* The Society for Research into Higher Education and OU Press, Buckingham.

Bolton, G. (2001) *Reflective Practice. Writing and Professional Development.* Paul Chapman Publishing Ltd, London.

Boud, D., Keogh, R. & Walker, D. (1985) *Reflection: Turning learning into experience.* Kogan Page, London.

Boyd, E.M. & Fales, A.W. (1983) Reflective learning: key to learning from experience. *Journal of Humanistic Psychology,* **23** (2), 99–117.

Brockbank, A. & McGill, I. (1998) *Facilitating Reflective Learning in Higher Education.* Society for Research in Higher Education and OU Press, Buckingham.

Burnard, P. (1995) Nurse educators' perceptions of reflection and reflective practice: a report of a descriptive study. *Journal of Advanced Nursing,* **21**, 1167–74.

Burns, S. & Bulman, C. (eds) (2000) *Reflective Practice. The Growth of the Professional Practitioner,* 2nd edn. Blackwell Science, Oxford.

Clarke, B., James, C. & Kelly, J. (1996) Reflective practice: reviewing the issues and refocusing the debate. *International Journal of Nursing Studies* **33** (20), 181–89.

Clarke, D.J. & Graham, M. (1996) Reflective practice, the use of reflective diaries by experienced registered nurses. *Nursing Review,* **15** (1), 26–9.

Clinton, M. (1998) On reflection in action: unaddressed issues in refocusing the debate in reflective practice. *International Journal of Nursing Practice*, 4 (30), 197–203.

Cottingham, J. (1997) *Descartes Philosophy of the Mind*. Phoenix, London.

Davies, C., Welham, V., Glover A. & Jones L. (1999) Teaching in practice. *Nursing Standard*, 13 (35), 33–9.

Day, J.M. (ed) (1994) *Plato's Meno in Focus*. Routledge, London.

Dewey, J. (1933) *How We Think. A restatement of the relation of reflective thinking to the educative process*. DC Heath. Massachusetts.

Duke, S. & Appleton, J. (2000) The use of reflection in a palliative care programme: a quantitative study of reflective skills over an academic year. *Journal of Advanced Nursing*, 32(6), 1557–68.

Durgahee, T. (1996) Promoting reflection in postgraduate nursing: a theoretical model. *Nurse Education Today*, 16, 419–26.

Eraut, M. (1994) *Developing Professional Knowledge and Competence*. Falmer Press, London.

FitzGerald, M. & Chapman, Y. (2000) Theories of Reflection for Learning. In: *Reflective Practice. The Growth of the Professional Practitioner* (eds S. Burns & C. Bulman), 2nd edn. Blackwell Science, Oxford.

Fonteyn, M.E. & Cahill, M. (1998) The use of clinical logs to improve nursing students' metacognition: a pilot study. *Journal of Advanced Nursing*, 28(1), 149–54.

Francis, D., Owens, J. & Tollefson, J. (1998) 'It comes together at the end': the impact of a one-year subject in nursing inquiry on philosophies of nursing. *Nursing Inquiry*, 5, 268–78.

Friere, P. (1972) *Pedagogy of the Oppressed*. Herder and Herder, New York.

Ghaye, Y. & Lilyman, S. (2000) *Reflection: Principles and practice for healthcare professionals*. Mark Allen Publishing Ltd, London.

Gibbs, G. (1988) *Learning by Doing. A Guide to Teaching and Learning Methods*. Oxford Polytechnic, Oxford.

Glaze, J. (2001a) Reflection as a transforming process: student advanced nurse practitioners' experiences on developing reflective skills as part of an MSc programme. *Journal of Advanced Nursing*, 34 (5) 639–47.

Glaze, J. (2001b) Stages in coming to terms with reflection: student advanced nurse practitioners' perceptions of their reflective journeys. *Journal of Advanced Nursing*, 37 (3), 265–72.

Goodman, J. (1984) Reflection and teacher education: A case study and theoretical analysis. *Interchange*, 15 (3), 9–26.

Graham, I.W. (2000) Reflective practice and its role in mental health nurses' practice development: a year long study. *Journal of Psychiatric and Mental Health Nursing*, 7, 109–17.

Green, A.J. & Holloway, D.G. (1997) Using a phenomenological research technique to examine student nurses' understandings of experiential teaching and learning: a critical review of methodological issues. *Journal of Advanced Nursing*, 26, 1013–1019.

Greenwood, J. (1998) The role of reflection in single and double loop learning. *Journal of Advanced Nursing* 27 (5), 1048–53.

Hallett, C.E. (1997) Learning through reflection in the community: the relevance of Schön's theories of coaching to nursing education. *International Journal of Nursing Studies*, 34 (2), 103–10.

Hart, G., Clinton, M., Edwards, H., Evans, K., Lunney, P., Posner, N., Tooth, B., Weir, D. & Ryan, Y. (2000) Accelerated professional development and peer consultation: Two strategies for continuing professional education for nurses. *The Journal of Continuing Education in Nursing*, 31 (1), 28–37.

Hayes, J. (1998) Learning from practice: Developing the reflective skills of forensic psychiatric nurses. *Psychiatric Care*, **5**(1), 30–33.

Heath, H. (1998) Paradigm dialogues and dogma: finding a place for research, nursing models and reflective practice. *Journal of Advanced Nursing* **28** (2), 288–94.

Hyrkas, K., Tarkka, M.T. & Paunonen-Ilmonen, M. (2001) Teacher candidates' reflective teaching and learning in a hospital setting – changing the pattern of practical training: a challenge to growing into teacher hood. *Journal of Advanced Nursing*, **33** (4), 503–11.

James, C.R. & Clarke, B.A. (1994) Reflective practice in nursing: issues and implications for nursing education *Nurse Education Today*, **14**, 82–90.

Jarvis, P. (1983) *Professional Education*. Croom Helm, London.

Jasper, M.A. (1999) Nurse's perceptions of the value of written reflection. *Nurse Education Today*, **19**, 452–63.

Johns, C. (1993) Professional supervision. *Journal of Nursing Management*, 1, 9–18.

Johns, C. (1994) Guided reflection. In: *Reflective Practice in Nursing. The Growth of the Professional Practitioner* (eds A. Palmer, S. Burns & C. Bulman). Blackwell Science, Oxford.

Johns, C. (1995a) The value of reflective practice for nursing. *Journal of Clinical Nursing*, **4**, 23–30.

Johns, C. (1995b) Framing learning through reflection within Carper's fundamental ways of knowing in nursing. *Journal of Advanced Nursing*, **22**, 226–34.

Johns, C. (2000) *Becoming a Reflective Practitioner. A reflective and holistic approach to clinical nursing, practice development and clinical supervision*. Blackwell Science, Oxford.

Johns, C. & Freshwater, D. (1998) *Transforming Nursing Through Reflective Practice*. Blackwell Publishing, Oxford.

Kember, D., Jones, A., Loke, A., McKay, J., Sinclair, K., Harrison, T., Webb, C., Wong, F., Wong, M., Yan, P.W. & Yeung, E. (1996) Developing curricula to encourage students to write reflective journals. *Educational Action Research* **4** (3), 329–48.

Kim, H.S. (1999) Critical reflective inquiry for knowledge development in nursing practice. *Journal of Advanced Nursing*, **29** (5), 1205–12.

Landeen, J., Byrne, C. & Brown, B. (1995) Exploring the lived experiences of psychiatric nursing students through self-reflective journals. *Journal of Advanced Nursing*, **21**, 878–85.

Liimatainen, L., Poskiparta, M., Karhila, P. & Sjogren, A. (2001) The development of reflective learning in the context of health counseling and health promotion during nurse education. *Journal of Advanced Nursing*, **34**(5), 648–58.

McCaugherty, D. (1991) The use of a teaching model to promote reflection and the experiential integration of theory and practice in first-year student nurses: an action research project. *Journal of Advanced Nursing*, **16**, 534–43.

McMahon, R. & Pearson, A. (eds) (1998) *Nursing as Therapy*, 2nd edn. Stanley Thornes, Cheltenham.

Mesirow, J. (1981) A critical theory of adult learning and education. *Adult Education*, **32** (1), 3–24.

Mountford, B. & Rogers, L. (1996) Using individual and group reflection in and on assessment as a tool for effective learning. *Journal of Advanced Nursing*, 24, 1127–34.

Page, S. & Meerabeau, L. (2000) Achieving change through reflective practice: closing the loop. *Nurse Education Today*, 20, 365–72.

Paget, T. (2001) Reflective practice and clinical outcomes: practitioners' views on how reflective practice has influenced their clinical practice. *Journal of Clinical Nursing*, **10**, 204–14.

Paterson, J.G. & Zderad, L.T. (1988) *Humanistic Nursing*. National League for Nursing, New York.

Platzer, H., Blake, D. & Ashford, D. (2000a) Barriers to learning from reflection: a study of the use of group work with post-registration students. *Journal of Advanced Nursing*, **31** (5), 1001–8.

Platzer, H., Blake, D. & Ashford, D. (2000b) An evaluation of process and outcomes from learning through reflective practice groups on a post-registration nursing course. *Journal of Advanced Nursing*, **31** (3), 689–95.

Polanyi, M. (1967) *The Tacit Dimension*. Doubleday, New York.

Powell, J. (1989) The reflective practitioner in nursing. *Journal of Advanced Nursing*, **14**, 824–32.

Reed, J. & Ground, I. (1997) *Philosophy for Nursing*. Arnold, London.

Reid, B. (1993) 'But we're doing it already!' Exploring a response to the concept of reflective practice in order to improve its facilitation. *Nurse Education Today*, **13**, 305–9.

Richardson, G. & Maltby, H. (1995) Reflection on practice: enhancing student learning. *Journal of Advanced Nursing*, **22**, 235–42.

Riley-Doucet, C. & Wilson, S. (1997) A three-step method of self-reflection using reflective journal writing. *Journal of Advanced Nursing*, **25**, 964–8.

Rogers, C. (1983) *Freedom to Learn for the 80s*. Merrill, Columbus, Ohio.

Rolfe, G., Freshwater, D. & Jasper, M. (2001) *Critical Reflection for Nursing and the Helping Professions; a user's guide*. Palgrave Macmillan, London.

Ryle, G. (1963) *The Concept of the Mind*. Penguin, Harmondsworth.

Ryle, G. (1979) *On Thinking*. Blackwell Publishing, Oxford.

Saylor, C. (1990) Reflection and professional education: art, science and competency. *Nurse Educator*, **15** (2), 8–11.

Scanlan, J.M., Dean Care, W. & Udod, S. (2002) Unraveling the unknowns of reflection in classroom teaching. *Journal of Advanced Nursing* 38(2), 136–43.

Schön, D.A. (1983) *The Reflective Practitioner*. Basic Books. Harper Collins, San Francisco.

Schön, D.A. (1987) *Educating the Reflective Practitioner*. Jossey Bass, San Francisco.

Schon, D.A. (1992) *The Reflective Practitioner*, 2nd edn. Jossey Bass, San Francisco.

Shields, E. (1995) Reflection and learning in student nurses. *Nurse Education Today*, **15**, 452–8.

Smith, A. (1998) Learning about reflection. *Journal of Advanced Nursing*, **28** (4), 891–8.

Snowball, J., Ross, K. & Murphy, K. (1994) Illuminating dissertation supervision through reflection. *Journal of Advanced Nursing*, **19**, 1234–40.

Sorrell, J.M., Brown, H.N., Cipriano Silva, M. & Kohlenberg, F.M. (1997) Use of writing portfolios for interdisciplinary assessment of critical thinking outcomes of nursing students. *Nursing Forum*, **32** (4), 12–24.

Spencer, N. & Newell, R. (1999) The use of brief written educational material to promote reflection amongst trained nurses: a pilot study. *Nurse Education Today*, **19**, 347–56.

Stoddart, B., Cope, P., Inglis, B., McIntosh, C. & Hislop, S. (1996) Student reflective groups at a Scottish College of Nursing. *Nursing Education Today*, **16**, 437–42.

Suhre, C.J.M. & Harskamp, E.G. (2001) Teaching planning and reflection in nurse education. *Nurse Education Today*, **21**, 373–81.

Teekman, B. (2000) Exploring reflective thinking in nursing practice. *Journal of Advanced Nursing*, 31(5), 1125–35.

UKCC (1994) The future of professional practice. The council's standards for education and practice following registration. United Kingdom Central Council for Nursing and Midwifery, London.

UKCC (1996) PREP and you – your guide to profiling. *Register*, **17**, 7–10.

Van Manen, M. (1977) Linking ways of knowing with ways of being practical. *Curriculum Inquiry*, **6** (3), 205–28.

Wallace, D. (1996) Experiential learning and critical thinking in nursing. *Nursing Standard*, **10** (31), 43–7.

Wittgenstein, L. (1967) *Philosophical Investigations*. Blackwell Publishing, Oxford.

Wong, F.K.Y., Loke, A.Y.L., Wong, M., Tse, H., Kan, E. & Kember, D. (1997) An action research study into the development of nurses as reflective practitioners. *Journal of Nursing Education*, **36** (10), 476–81.

Chapter 2

Developing Underlying Skills in the Move Towards Reflective Practice

Sue Atkins

Introduction

This chapter is based on an assumption that there are certain skills underlying the development and use of reflective practice. During the past ten years there has been much discussion and debate within nursing and other health care education literature about the nature of reflection and how reflective practice may be facilitated in professional courses (Clarke *et al.* 1996; Greenwood 1998; Burton 2000). A number of small research studies have been undertaken to investigate reflective learning, for example Durgahee (1998), Jasper (1999) and Page and Meerabeau (2000). It is now widely understood that reflective practice is a process of learning and development through examining one's own practice including experiences, thoughts, feelings, actions and knowledge (Mezirow 1981; Brockbank & McGill 1998; Kim 1999; Bolton 2001). These and other authors emphasise that reflection involves reviewing one's own values, challenging assumptions and considering broader social, political and professional issues that are relevant but may be beyond personal practice experience. This is considered to be essential if reflection is to result in significant and positive social change, and what Argyris *et al.* (1985) and Greenwood (1998) refer to as double-loop learning.

An earlier review of key literature on reflection from the fields of education and critical social theory, suggested that the skills of self-awareness, description, critical analysis, synthesis and evaluation were necessary to engage in reflective practice (Atkins & Murphy 1993). The purpose of this chapter is to explore these skills, and present a series of exercises aimed at helping nurses and other health and social care professionals to examine, develop and refine their skills.

It is evident that the deliberate and systematic use of reflection as a learning tool in professional practice is a complex activity that needs to be consciously developed by pre and post-qualifying professionals over time (Burrows 1995; Duke & Appleton 2000; Glaze 2001). It is also widely acknowledged that the development of reflective learning and practice requires skilled, sensitive facilitation, and appropriate guidance and support from educators, supervisors and mentors (Brockbank & McGill 1998; Johns 2000; Paget 2001). A variety of approaches are used to facilitate reflection. These include the use of models and structured frameworks (Gibbs 1988; Johns 1996), reflective writing and the use of journals (Paterson 1995; Bolton 2001), engaging in reflective dialogue (Brockbank & McGill 1998; Bolton 2001), and the use of action learning sets (McGill & Beaty 2001).The intention of the skills-based approach presented in this chapter is to complement these approaches.

A series of exercises is presented for use by practitioners and facilitators, with a separate section devoted to each skill. The meaning of the skill is defined and explored, highlighting its relevance for both professional practice and academic work. The importance of each skill for reflective practice is justified with reference to key theories and recent research. The exercises enable participants to practise the skills of reflection alone, with a colleague or friend and within a group. The importance of combining individual and group activity in the development of reflective learning is supported by research studies, for example Durgahee (1996) and Wong *et al.* (1997). In particular, the value of engaging in reflective dialogue with others in order to achieve deeper levels of reflection is apparent.

The importance of underlying skills

An examination of the nature and process of reflective practice, as discussed by key and influential theorists, for example Mezirow (1981), Boud et al (1985) and Schön (1991), suggests that there are underlying skills involved in reflective practice. The skills of self-awareness, description, critical analysis, synthesis and evaluation are implicit in the models and theories of these authors. For example, in Boud *et al.*'s (1985) analysis of the reflective process, the need to attend to feelings and attitudes, in particular making use of positive feelings and dealing with negative feelings, is apparent throughout and requires self-awareness. The stages labelled as 'Association', 'Integration', 'Validation' and 'Appropriation' involve varying degrees of critical analysis, synthesis and evaluation. Similarly, if one takes Mesirow's (1981) concept of reflectivity and studies its seven different dimensions or levels, it is clear that self-awareness is integral at all levels (see Chapter 9). The need for description, analysis, synthesis and evaluation becomes more evident when moving up the hierarchy from 'Discriminant' to 'Theoretical' reflectivity. Schön's (1991) analysis of the reflective practitioner's use of reflection-on-action and reflection-in-action implies the use of similar skills. More recently, the development of structured models and frameworks to guide reflective practice in nursing education makes the use of these skills more explicit (Johns 1996; Duke & Appleton 2000).

The importance of these underlying skills has been reinforced by a number of small-scale research projects that examine the development of reflection in students undertaking pre and post-qualifying nursing courses (Wong *et al.* 1997; Jasper 1999; Duke & Appleton 2000; Glaze 2001; Paget 2001). Jasper's (1999) grounded theory study identified reflective writing as an important strategy for developing self-awareness and critical analysis. Duke and Appleton's (2000) quantitative study demonstrated that palliative care students' reflective skills developed over an academic year, and that the higher level skills necessary for critical reflection were harder to develop and took longer to achieve. In Glaze's (2001) exploratory study of student advanced nurse practitioners' experiences of developing reflective skills, the practitioners describe their deepening self-awareness, greater critical analysis abilities, especially in relation to socio-political issues, and their efforts at synthesis and evaluation through attempts to empower colleagues and bring about changes in practice.

It is interesting to note that there are similarities between skills underlying reflective practice and the skills required for academic work. With the exception of self-awareness, these underlying skills are the higher order cognitive or thinking skills identified within Bloom *et al*'s (1956) taxonomy of educational objectives. This taxonomy or hierarchy has guided and influenced the development of learning programmes, objectives and outcomes within higher education. Therefore, developing and refining these underlying skills may not only help to develop a more reflective style of practice, but may further the development of academic skills and ability to integrate theory with practice. This is especially important for people undertaking work-based learning and professional development courses.

Limitations of a skills-based approach to developing reflective practice

It is important to acknowledge the limitations of a skills-based exercise approach to developing reflective practice. Reflective practice skills are acquired and developed gradually through practice over time, rather than in any one course or package (see Chapter 8). While the exercises in this chapter involve reflecting on practice, frequently away from the clinical setting, it is important to acknowledge that reflective practice, most importantly, is a way of examining thoughts, feelings and actions while actually engaged in professional practice, as illustrated in Schön's (1991) work. Greenwood (1998) also emphasises the importance of reflection before action

People have individual styles of learning and may learn in different ways, depending on their personality, maturity and experience. Therefore, the extent to which individuals may find the skills-based approach to developing reflective practice presented in this chapter, to be helpful is likely to vary. Highly structured and staged approaches to developing skills for reflective practice may be more suitable for less experienced students on pre-registration programmes, as indicated by the work of Burrows (1995). It has been suggested by Bolton (2001) that the use of structured frameworks and exercises may be restrictive and counter-productive to the development of creativity in professional practice. Bolton (2001) advocates a less structured narrative approach whereby practitioners write freely about their practice experiences and share their writing within a facilitated group.

It is apparent that other skills, not addressed in this chapter, are also important, especially when engaging in reflection with other people. These include skills of active listening, empathy, assertiveness, supporting and challenging and the planning and management of change (Brockbank & McGill 1998; Durgahee 1998; Page & Meerabeau (2000). In particular, change management skills are important if the outcome of reflection is to have a positive impact on practice. It is recommended that readers consult some of the many texts available on change management, for example Burnes (2000) or Broome's (1998) practical guide.

Guidance on using the exercises in this chapter

Three types of exercises are presented:

- *On-your-own exercises*. It is recommended that about 15-30 minutes is spent on these exercises.
- *With-a-partner exercises*. These exercises may take approximately 30–60 minutes.
- *Group exercises*. These exercises may take between 30 and 90 minutes.

All exercises require a commitment of time and thought. Taking the exercises slowly over several weeks is recommended as the best approach. It will also be helpful to refer to the many examples and extracts of reflection within other chapters of this book.

Issues for facilitators

It is recommended that facilitators are educators or supervisors who are experienced and feel comfortable working with adult learners. Facilitators are reminded of the importance of role modelling, and that they need to be reflective practitioners themselves. There is a growing body of literature focusing on the development of the reflective teacher and the facilitation of reflective learning, including, for example, Scanlan and Chernomas (1997), Brockbank and McGill (1998) and Light and Cox (2001).

Facilitators may prepare themselves by following these guidelines:

- Review all exercises from a personal point of view, as well as from an educational perspective. If you have not had the opportunity to engage in the exercises as a participant prior to being a facilitator, it is recommended that you at least challenge yourself with the on-your-own exercises.
- Be prepared to role model or participate in all exercises. It is essential that the facilitator demonstrates an openness and willingness to share experiences. Reflecting on experiences may be seen as uncomfortable and risky by some participants. Facilitators may provide support and encouragement by example.
- Co-facilitation is suggested, where possible and depending on the size of the group. With more than one facilitator, participants can benefit by the increased accessibility of a facilitator. The facilitators can also benefit from the opportunity for ongoing dialogue and reflection with a peer.
- Bearing in mind the limitations of such a programme of exercises, and the fact that they are in no way intended to be comprehensive, facilitators should be prepared to guide participants to further appropriate resources.
- Normally, ground rules would need to be established when working with a group in this way.

Self-awareness

To be self-aware is to be conscious of one's character, including beliefs, values, qualities, strengths and limitations. It is about knowing oneself. Burnard (1992) distinguishes between the inner self, how one feels inside, and the outer self, the aspects that other people see, including appearance, verbal and non-verbal behaviour.

Self-awareness may be described as the foundation skill upon which reflective practice is built. It underpins the entire process of reflection because it enables people to see themselves in a particular situation and honestly observe how they have affected the situation and how the situation has affected them. Self-awareness enables a person to analyse her or his own feelings, beliefs and values, an essential part of the reflective process. It is evident from influential literature that it is the use of self-awareness and self or personal knowledge which differentiates reflective learning from other types of mental activity, for example logical thinking and problem solving (Mezirow 1981; Boud *et al.* 1985). All adult learners need to be self-aware. This enables them to take responsibility for identifying and responding to their learning needs, and to develop greater independence in initiating, planning, conducting and communicating work, whether in relation to formal study or professional lifelong learning.

It is also important, although obvious, to state that self-awareness is essential, not only for reflective learning but also for skilled professional nursing practice. In particular, knowledge of one's own beliefs, values and behaviour, and how these affect others, is essential for developing good interpersonal skills and building therapeutic relationships with patients.

In some ways, self-awareness is hard to avoid, as self-interest is part of human nature. However, developing an honest self-awareness is more complex. It is natural to want to see and portray oneself in the most favourable light. This desire, together with our own prejudices and assumptions, can sometimes interfere with the ability to take a more objective look at oneself. Being honest about oneself therefore requires courage, confidence, a certain degree of maturity, and the support of others. In particular, to develop and maintain an appropriate level of self-awareness in the work situation and for reflective practice requires substantial effort and mental energy. One is sometimes dealing with deeply held values and strong feelings which may be uncomfortable and anxiety provoking. There may, therefore, be times when one chooses to avoid the process, and when it is becomes more appropriate just to go home and relax. It is, however, important to bear in mind that identifying and releasing one's feelings, both positive and negative, is generally better for a person, provided that the time and place are appropriate. While a degree of personal insight and self-awareness is necessary to engage in reflective practice, it is also important to recognise that too much negative introspection and analysis can have an adverse effect. Therefore, there is a need to gain the right balance in any situation.

The following exercises aim to help you identify and clarify beliefs, values and feelings. There are also exercises enabling you to examine your motivation for developing a more reflective type of practice, and the degree to which you are open and receptive to new ideas. These factors have been identified as essential pre-requisites for reflective practice (Boud *et al.* 1985; Wong *et al*, 1997).

On-your-own exercise: clarifying values *15 min*

A personal value can be described by a statement that says what is important and significant to you as an individual. Describe three of your own values below by completing this sentence:

It is important to me that . . .
(1) . . .
(2) . . .
(3) . . .

With-a-partner exercise: exploring values *30 min*

- Are you clear and certain about what your values are? Give examples. Identify some values that are key for you.
- Do your values always guide your actions? Give examples of when they have done and when they have not.
- How did you acquire the key values in your life? Identify specific people or situations that have affected your values.

Go over the answers to these questions with a partner. Consider how you can become clearer about your own values.

Values perform an important function for everyone. They provide a clear framework for deciding upon a position and they provide a basis for action. Being clear about your values in professional practice is also important because it will help you to live with the results of your actions. What is interesting about values is that they are chosen but they are not necessarily consistent with one another.

On-your-own exercise: how motivated am I? *15 min*

Think about the reasons why you are developing and using reflection. Make a list of these.

You may have identified some good reasons. In addition to enabling you to develop and enhance your nursing practice, reflection is important within formal professional courses, and when profiling learning for professional registration purposes, for the assessment and accreditation of prior experiential learning (APEL) and for demonstrating work-based learning. If, however, you believe you have little to gain personally or professionally you may find it more difficult to devote the necessary time. There is always the possibility that this is not the right approach for you or that this is not the right time for you to undertake the exercises.

On-your-own exercise: am I open to new ideas?　*30 mins*

Identify from your professional practice a situation where a colleague introduced a change that would or did have implications for your own practice.

- Describe what the change was.
- What were the significant background factors to this change?
- What were your thoughts about it?
- Identify your feelings about the change.
- How receptive were you to the change? Why was this?
- What were your prejudices and biases?

This exercise may have highlighted two issues. First, change may not necessarily be for the better. It may be that you had negative feelings towards the change, and that this was because you did not see the change as in the best interests of the team or patients. It may be that you felt there was insufficient evidence to support the change. Second, you may find change in itself difficult. If so, you need to consider carefully the reasons why. Changes can make people feel insecure and unsettled. There may also be some times in your life when you are more receptive to change than at other times. It is, however, important to remember that openness to new ideas is necessary to be a reflective practitioner.

On-your-own exercise: your life map　*15–30 min*

On a large piece of paper draw a map or diagram that represents the background and history of your nursing practice or training. Include as much detail as possible. Putting your nursing practice into a picture format may seem awkward or difficult at first, but it will allow you to see your career from a very different perspective. Don't worry about drawing things correctly, just try to be creative.

　Include as many of the following events as possible:

- your starting point
- achievements
- joys
- sadnesses
- important people
- obstacles.

With-a-partner exercise: directions and destinations   *30–60 min*

Take turns explaining the map of your career in nursing or your experiences as a nursing student. Give as much detail as possible, so that your partner can understand your background.

When listening to your partner, pay close attention to the details. Ask questions to better understand your partner's experiences. Also listen for what is left out of your partner's story. Here are some questions you may want to use to probe a little deeper.

- Where are you on your map? How active or passive are you?
- Where are the strongest emotions on your map? What are these emotions? Have any emotionally strong experiences been left out?
- Are there any other people on your map? Who are they? Is anyone missing who should be there?
- Are there patients on your map? Why or why not?
- What takes up the most space on your map? Why do you think it does?
- Are there any empty spaces on your map? Should something else be included in those spaces? Is there any meaning in the emptiness?

Group exercise: looking for the cross-roads   *30-60 min*

All participants should post their 'maps' on the walls of the room. Without describing or analysing the maps, look for what is common:

- themes
- symbols
- depictions
- colour choices
- any developments or sequences (e.g. from left to right, bottom to top).

Given the fact that members of the group have lived through similar times and are engaged in the same profession, it is not surprising that there may be common areas. Value the shared experiences since they can bind the group together and also provide support. Look also for the differences between the 'maps'. These unique versions are valuable to the group in a different way in providing new perspectives.

Spend a few minutes talking about the experience of 'mapping'. Allow each participant a chance to answer the question:

- What was the biggest surprise or insight you got from your own or others' life maps?

Life maps remind us of the positive aspects of our careers, but will also bring to mind the low points or sadnesses that we have experienced. Be prepared to support members of the group who need it.

Description

To describe something, whether it be a person, an object, a situation or an abstract concept or idea, is to state its characteristics or appearance without expressing a judgement. A descriptive account is usually in spoken or written form, but may also be in other forms, such as a painting or sculpture.

In appreciating the qualities and power of good description, examples of excellent descriptive accounts are widely available within English literature. In particular, the reader is referred to Styles and Moccia's (1993) anthology *On Nursing: a Literary Celebration* which contains many rich descriptive accounts of nursing, and people's experiences of health and illness. In professional practice, good descriptive abilities are necessary when communicating with colleagues about patients and for writing clear and accurate patient progress notes.

When using reflection-on-practice, description is the skill with which you recollect the important events and features of your practice. Good description is about giving a clear, accurate and comprehensive account of a situation. The account will include the following key elements: significant background factors (the context), the events as they unfolded in the situation, what you were thinking at the time, how you were feeling at the time, and the outcome of the situation. Your description should reconstruct the situation, to enable someone who was not there to understand the situation from your position. What you are trying to do is paint a clear, vivid, colourful picture that then allows you and possibly others to review the situation.

Some people are gifted with the skill of description while others struggle more to find the most appropriate words to express themselves. A full vocabulary is necessary to be able to describe situations accurately, but at the same time there is a need to avoid the use of jargon and terminology which the reader or listener may not understand. It is also important to discriminate between relevant and irrelevant information. A good descriptive account, therefore, demonstrates a full and clear understanding of the relevant and important issues, and is well structured and concise.

Within a piece of written reflection, or when engaging in reflection with another person or a group, it is also important to achieve a balance between description of the situation and the analytical processes which follow. In particular, when undertaking work for academic purposes, it is often the higher order thinking skills of analysis and evaluation that are most valued. However, it may be more difficult to engage in these critical thinking processes without good underlying descriptive skills.

On-your-own exercise: the power of description   *30 min.*

Choose a page of literature from a favourite text, for example a novel, autobiography or poem. Read it carefully. When you feel that you are really familiar with the passage, write down:

- key elements of the description which capture the essence of the situation
- important words or phrases which facilitated your understanding.

It is important to consider what the elements of good description are. If you are able to incorporate these into your writing, you are more likely to give the comprehensive account that enables you to demonstrate your learning through experience. A good piece of description paints a clear and vivid picture of a unique situation. It enables the reader to understand the situation from the writer's perspective. The description contains details that capture not only the significant background factors, but also bring to life these situations through the use of carefully selected words.

On-your-own exercise: I remember when...   *30 min*

Identify a work situation in which you were involved recently. The situation might include one or more of the following features:

- you felt that your actions made a real difference to a patient or group of patients
- it went unusually well
- it did not go as planned
- it was very ordinary and typical of your professional practice
- it captures the essence of what your professional practice is about.

Take some time to think about the situation. Bearing in mind the features of good description, write down as many of the details that you can remember. You need to avoid using the *specific* names of people or places involved, to preserve anonymity and confidentiality. Be sure to include information on the following:

- where and when the situation occurred
- who was involved in the situation
- the specific circumstances of the care provided/not provided
- how you felt about the situation at the time
- what you did at the time of the situation
- how you coped after the situation
- what you thought and felt about the situation at a later time.

With-a-partner exercise: 'Let me tell you about...'   *30–60 min*

Using your notes from the on-your-own exercise, tell your partner of your experience. Don't be limited by what you wrote. Use your notes as a starting point. When listening to your partner, pay close attention to the details. Ask questions to better understand your partner's experiences. Also listen for what is left out of your partner's story. You may want to probe a little deeper. In telling this story did you talk more about what you felt, thought and did, or did you describe the actions and attitudes of others?

To facilitate another person's understanding of a situation, you need to give all the relevant factors in enough detail. A common problem may be that because you were involved in the situation, you may omit certain details that you have taken for granted. You may also find it difficult to recall all of the key factors in the situation because you have to rely on your memory. It is likely that the situations you will be most able to describe are those that occurred more recently. Sometimes it is important that you can describe situations from your nursing practice, even though they may have occurred some time ago. Keeping a diary that records and describes events in your professional practice may therefore enhance your descriptive abilities.

On-your-own exercise: describing feelings *30 min*

Think of a situation in your professional practice where the outcomes were not what you expected or you felt uncomfortable about them. Describe the situation using the elements of good description, and then answer the following questions:

- Does your description capture the essence of the situation?
- Does what you have written describe your feelings accurately and truthfully?

It is not always easy to describe the feelings you have. Some people find it easier to describe their thoughts about a situation rather than their feelings. When feelings are strong, for example when we are very happy or very upset, they tend to be easier to acknowledge. However, in any situation there are likely to be feelings beneath the surface that may need more detailed exploration to uncover. Some people find it easier to express feelings than others. If this is true for you, you need to consider some of the reasons why this might be the case. It is, however, generally believed that we are better off identifying and releasing feelings (Boyd & Fales 1983; Brockbank & McGill 1998).

On-your-own exercise: judging your description *30 min*

This exercise is designed to enable you to judge how effective your skills of description are. Take the description you wrote in one of the previous exercises. Using the rating scale below, award yourself up to five points for each statement. The maximum score would be 15.

- My description captures the situation accurately.
- My feelings were accurately and honestly reported.
- The key elements are concisely presented.

Look at your score. What were your particular strengths and weaknesses? Some people find it easier to describe facts rather than feelings. An awareness of the difficulties you have will allow you to focus on these and build skills further. If your score fell below 6, you may need to consider repeating these exercises.

Group exercise: my career – the film *30–90 min*

Having had an opportunity to get an overview of your career or background, as well as a close-up look at a significant incident, you are now in the position of being able to step back for a 'big screen' picture. Ask each member of the group to consider the statement below:

Contd.

- If I were to make a film version of this episode of my career, it would most appropriately be titled...

Feel free to borrow or improvise from existing films or to make up your own title. Write the answer on a Post-it Note or index card. Ask each member to paste their film title on to a large piece of paper or poster board in the room. As people put up their titles they should explain the reasons for their choice. People may group their titles with those of a similar nature (adventure films, action, disaster, etc.).

Imagining our careers as films may at first seem trivial, but it can be fun! It also allows the imaginative parts of our brains to put together the disparate pieces of our life into an image that is easier to understand and describe to others.

Critical analysis

Critical analysis is a key skill for both reflective practice and academic work. Analysis involves the separation of a whole into its component parts. To analyse something, whether an object, a set of ideas or a situation, is to undertake a detailed examination of the structure or constituent parts or elements and ask questions about them, in order to more fully understand their nature and how the parts relate to and influence each other. The term 'critical' introduces a further dimension to analysis, in that judgements are made about the strengths and weaknesses of the different parts, as well as of the whole. Being critical does have some negative connotations when it is used in everyday life, in that it is a term often associated with finding fault. However, engaging in critical analysis, or undertaking a critique of something, is a positive and constructive process, because it is about identifying strengths as well as weaknesses. Examples of using critical analysis in professional practice include assessing the needs of an individual patient, as well as making a broader contribution to service and policy development.

   Some authors emphasise critical analysis as a rational, linear, problem-solving process grounded in the scientific approach (Siegal 1988; Fisher 1995). However, the more widely accepted view appears to be that critical analysis and critical thinking involve an emotional dimension (Brookfield 1987; Daly 1998; Light & Cox 2001). Acknowledging and analysing beliefs, values and feelings is a fundamental and important part if the outcome of reflective practice is to have a positive effect on professional learning, practice development and the quality of patient care. As a health care professional, the situations you are involved in may be unique, and therefore the knowledge that you need in order to understand and solve problems in practice will depend on the individual components of the situation and the broader context. It is also important to recognise that any situation will be influenced by your own feelings, attitudes and behaviour. When engaging in reflective practice, therefore, the skill of critical analysis involves the following activities:

- identifying and illuminating existing knowledge of relevance to the situation
- exploring feelings about the situation and the influence of these

- identifying and challenging assumptions made
- imagining and exploring alternative courses of action (Broc

Identifying existing knowledge

The knowledge required for understanding a specific situation tified and scrutinised. You may find that in order to shed light or need to search for and examine other knowledge that at first may not have seemed relevant. It is therefore important that you identify the types and sources of knowledge that you use in your professional nursing practice. This is about raising questions such as 'what do we know?' and 'how do we know it?'

Professional knowledge, and nursing knowledge in particular, has been classified in a number of ways (Carper 1978, 1992; Higgs & Titchen 2000). While recognising that any classification is artificial, and different types of knowledge are interdependent, it is sometimes helpful to refer to a framework or classification when examining one's own knowledge. In western philosophy, a common distinction has been between propositional knowledge or 'know-that', which is theoretical knowledge and knowledge generated through research, and non-propositional knowledge or 'know-how', which consists of personal knowledge, practical skills and expertise (Polanyi 1958; Higgs & Titchen 2000). The work of Carper (1978, 1992) has been influential within nursing theory, and is used in some frameworks for reflection, for example Johns (1995). Carper identifies four fundamental patterns of knowing from an analysis of the structure of nursing knowledge:

- Empirical knowledge is the factual, descriptive and theoretical knowledge, often developed through research.
- Aesthetic knowledge is knowledge gained more subjectively, through unique and particular situations, and is sometimes referred to as the art of nursing.
- Personal knowledge refers to knowledge of self, used for example in building therapeutic relationships with patients and in helping them cope with illness.
- Ethical knowledge is concerned with understandings and judgements of what is right, wrong or ought to be done in different situations.

Therefore, engaging in a thorough critical analysis involves analysing one's knowledge and where necessary, actively seeking out the ideas, theories and research of others.

Exploring feelings related to the situation

In reflective practice, it is necessary to gain an appropriate balance between the analysis of knowledge and thoughts, and the analysis of feelings. It is also important to focus on positive feelings as well as trying to deal with negative feelings, in order for the process to be constructive (Boud *et al.* 1985). What needs to be remembered, however, is that the overall purpose of reflection is to contribute to improvements and further developments in patient care. It is the feelings and experiences of patients that are of central concern. Therefore, analysis of one's eelings may be a process which one engages in only so far as it affects and luminates practice situations, and enhances learning from those situations.

Identifying and challenging assumptions

Identifying assumptions is about recognising when information is taken for granted or presented as fact without the supporting evidence. It is about not taking things at face value. When analysing a situation it may be helpful to ask questions like 'what is being taken for granted here?' and 'how do I know that I've got an accurate picture of the situation?' It may be easy to carry on through working and personal lives with the same set of assumptions, beliefs and values about oneself, about nursing, and about the health care practice in general. However, there is a need to challenge these assumptions regularly, and to question where they have come from. Challenging the relevance of the context is particularly important. Everything that happens does so within a certain context, so it is important to be able to examine the ideas of people from different backgrounds, and consider them within the context of our own. Assuming that ideas and practices which work in one context can automatically be carried to another can cause problems. Examples of such difficulties have sometimes been evident in attempts to apply North American nursing models and health care systems to nursing in the UK.

When identifying and challenging assumptions, it is important to be sceptical of claims to universal truth. Simply because a practice has existed for a long time does not mean that it is most appropriate. Just because an idea is accepted by others does not mean that one has to believe in its innate truth, without first checking its correspondence with one's own experience (Brookfield 1987).

Challenging the assumptions underlying one's own ideas and those of others can be an uncomfortable experience and may involve asking awkward questions. It is therefore important to raise awareness, prompt, nurture and encourage the process without making people feel threatened.

Imagining and exploring alternative courses of action

Central to this is the idea of constantly looking for new ways of thinking and new ways of doing things. Such new ways of living allow for creativity and growth as opposed to routine and stasis. You could ask yourself the following questions: 'Do I still work in the same way as I did two years ago? Is that appropriate? What, if anything, do I want to do about that?' This aspect of critical analysis also requires one to look at perspectives other than one's own.

On-your-own exercise: analysing your knowledge   *30 min*

Take a situation previously described. Think about the knowledge that has enabled you to understand the situation. Write a detailed account of relevant knowledge and indicate the sources of the knowledge.

Some of the knowledge you have used is likely to have been gained through personal experience. Remember that while this is a useful and valid way of gaining knowledge, you need to explore the extent to which this knowledge helps you understand the situation. Some knowledge may have been gained through 'trial and error'. It is particularly important to question this knowledge and what its value is. In the climate of evidence-based professional practice, formal knowledge must be a key source of knowledge, and it is important that your account contains research-based knowledge where appropriate. If you have been unable to identify any formal sources of knowledge, it may be that you need to do some further thinking and reading. Group or cultural knowledge can be more difficult to identify, as this knowledge is often implicit in everyday practice. It may be taken for granted or be bound up in the assumptions that underlie your practice. It is important that you explore any assumptions made.

With-a-partner exercise: discussing your knowledge   *30–60 min*

Ask a partner to read the situation you described previously. Discuss together the knowledge which each of you considers is relevant to understanding the situation:

- Was the knowledge that your partner identified the same or different from yours?
- If different, explore the reasons why.
- Agree with your partner which knowledge was most important for understanding the situation.
- Try to identify together any new knowledge that would be relevant to the situation, and suggest alternative knowledge which may give new insights.

On-your-own exercise: analysing your feelings   *30 min*

Take a situation described previously. Identify any excerpts that involved feelings. Read through the excerpt carefully. See whether you have identified your feelings where appropriate. If not, why not? Try to explore honestly why you felt the way you did.

If necessary, try again to identify your feelings. Taking the relevant excerpt, think carefully and identify the feelings which were important in that situation. This may include feelings you had within the situation and about it, the feelings you had at the time and the feelings you have now.

Answer the following questions:

- Why did you feel the way you did?
- What are the relevant elements that made you feel that way?
- Was there anything relevant in your past experiences which led you to feel the way you did?

With-a-partner exercise: talking about feelings   *30 min*

Talk through your feelings with someone you trust.

Reflective practice does involve an analysis of feelings, and without this understanding you may miss real opportunities in your experience to learn about yourself. Increasing self-awareness and the ability to analyse your feelings will give you insights that may enhance your professional practice. While analysis of feelings is difficult, if you have not been able to undertake this exercise, you need to consider carefully the reasons why.

On-your-own exercise: 'One way of looking at it.'   *30 min*

Critically analyse a situation previously described, from as many different perspectives as possible. Try to imagine the point of view of patients, colleagues and other people who were involved in the situation.

With-a-partner exercise: 'Different ways of looking at it.'   *30–60 min*

Practise taking opposing opinions on the situation presented in the previous exercise. Try defending a perspective that is not your own. Support your views with formal knowledge or theory where possible.

Frequently health care professionals operate from substantially different viewpoints. When a dilemma presents itself, people react differently based on their beliefs and principles. The resulting conflict can be both upsetting and baffling. It may be hard sometimes to understand how equally concerned caregivers can have opposing opinions. However, in the climate of interprofessional working it is becoming increasingly important to understand and respect the values of others.

Group exercise: the great debate   *30–90 min*

Divide the group into several teams, depending on the size of the group. Each team should identify and will then represent a key theory used in professional nursing practice. The teams should be asked to debate the following question:

● What theory provides the most value to health care providers?

Team members should work together to develop their arguments. One or two members of the team should be selected as spokespersons for the group.
Round 1 – each team is allowed five minutes to state the reason why their theory is the most useful to health care providers.
Round 2 – each team is given five minutes to state the reasons why the other theories presented are inadequate in meeting the needs of health care providers.
Success of the teams will be based on the clarity of their communication and arguments.

Synthesis

Synthesis is defined by the Oxford Dictionary as 'the process or result of building up separate elements, especially ideas, into a connected and coherent whole'. It could be described as the opposite of analysis.

Synthesis is about the artistry of professional practice, and about being creative. It may involve original thinking. At a fundamental level of practice, devising a patient care plan is an example of the synthesis of information from a variety of different sources. A good care plan is unique to the particular patient and is dynamic.

When using reflection, synthesis is the ability to integrate new knowledge, feelings or attitudes with previous knowledge, feelings or attitudes. This is necessary in order to develop a fresh insight or a new perspective on a situation and therefore to learn from it. The skill of synthesis is necessary, therefore, in order to achieve a satisfactory outcome from reflection. This may include the clarification of an issue, the development of a new attitude or way of thinking about something, the resolution of a problem, a change in behaviour or a decision. Such changes may be small or large. New knowledge may potentially be generated and original ideas or fresh ways of approaching problems or answering questions may be developed. Synthesis involves making choices with regard to relating new ideas to one's past beliefs and values. This may not necessarily be an easy process, depending on the scope of adjustment being made. You may choose not to incorporate new ideas and instead maintain the old ones; this is not necessarily right or wrong. Changing old ideas should not be done indiscriminately. The important point is that the choice is an informed decision.

The skill of synthesis can be a difficult one. Listening to the way others have put the pieces together in relation to different situations may be helpful at this point.

On-your-own exercise: 'Dear Friend . . .'   *30 min*

Take some time to think about what you have learned from the previous exercises and write a letter to a friend, real or imagined, telling of the changes you have experienced. Be sure to include some of the following:

- Give an update on yourself and your self-awareness. Has it changed? What did you learn by mapping out your career and talking it over with a partner?
- Describe one of the situations that you believe has most influenced your practice.
- Include information about any knowledge or theory you believe has most relevance to your practice.
- Finish off by writing about what you intend to do differently in identifying and handling some of the issues you encounter in your practice.

With-a-partner exercise: spotlight on you   *30–60 min*

In addition to the written reflections that you have undertaken during these exercises, you now have the opportunity to make a video. By recording your thoughts on video you will be able to hear and see yourself express your views about your nursing practice. You will also be able to use the video recording as a yardstick against which to measure your professional growth in the future. On completion, the videotape will be yours alone. There will be no need to share it with anyone other than your partner for the exercises. However, you may choose to show it to a facilitator, friend, family member or mentor, or you may decide to view it again in the privacy of your own home. You have done all the preparation for this experience in the previous exercises. There is no need to use notes or check your readings. Your partner will prompt you with the questions listed below:

1. Tell me a little bit about who you are. (Remember the information that you put in the map of your career. You may wish to add to that information.)
2. Think of a meaningful incident in your professional career. Tell me:
    - what your role was
    - what were the choices that you had
    - what was the choice you made
    - how you felt about your choice.
    (You do not need to use the incident you described previously in the section on description. Discussion of that incident may have brought to mind other situations that you have faced in practice.)
3. Where and what type of work would you like to see yourself doing? What changes and improvements would you make in the way you approach and handle the issues that you face?
    Try answering these questions in the following time frames:
    - one-year goals
    - five-year goals
    - end of practice goals.

The idea of videotaping yourself may be intimidating. You may wonder if it is necessary. One of the reasons you are strongly encouraged to videotape yourself in this session is that it allows you the rare opportunity of seeing yourself. Unlike home videos in which the emphasis may be on how you look, this video will focus on what you say and how you say it. You will be able to see yourself as others see you and gain a different perspective on yourself. A video, unlike a written account, is more spontaneous, allowing you to say what is on your mind without worrying about punctuation or grammar.

Group exercise: the video experience   *30–90 min*

Looking at oneself in pictures or on videotape can be an unnerving experience that many approach with fear and others simply avoid. Having just created a videotape of yourself, it is a good time to discuss the experience. As a group, try to take a look at the benefits and risks of having been videotaped. Each participant should independently write down all the advantages and all the disadvantages that videotaping presents. Then going around the room, each participant should mention one plus and one minus about the

Contd.

video that has not yet been mentioned by the other participants. Keep circling the group until all the items on everyone's list have been mentioned.

Listing all the pluses and minuses on a flip chart will give participants a 'master list'. Reviewing this complete list will allow individuals, as well as the group, to make a final decision on the merits of videotaping. You may find that this discussion will give you new ideas on how you can review and use your videotape in the future.

Evaluation

Evaluation is the ability to make a judgement about the value of something. It entails a 'looking back'.

Judgements are often made with reference to predefined criteria or standards, for example when assessing the value of a research report, when determining whether or not a patient has achieved certain goals or when monitoring and auditing the extent to which targets have been achieved within health services. Evaluation is a high level skill in both reflective practice and traditional academic work. Unfortunately, the idea of evaluation can make people feel uncomfortable, because of its association with examinations, performance appraisals and other assessments. The fear of being judged badly may make people want to avoid it altogether.

Self-assessment or evaluation is a personal process in which one examines oneself, frequently over time. This is an important component of reflective practice and professional education. While we can receive input from others and include their observations and opinions, ultimately one must judge oneself. People can frequently be their own toughest critics. Evaluation should not be self-torture for past problems. Rather it is future orientated, for example it may involve finding discrepancies between what is said and needed, and what is actually done, in order to make necessary changes. Autobiographies often contain interesting examples of self-evaluation, showing how people look back on their lives.

On-your-own exercise: listening to yourself and others   *15–30 min*

Play back your own or, with permission, your partner's video. Listen to what you or your partner say on the videotape and take notes on the following:

- beliefs/values
- problems to overcome
- goals for the future.

With-a-partner exercise: learning from the past and looking to the future   *30–60 min*

Review with your partner the notes that you have taken about the video. Ask your partner if they agree with each of the items you have put into the categories of beliefs/ values, problems to overcome, and goals for the future.

Contd.

After the discussion with your partner, change any of the items if necessary. Use the rest of the time with your partner identifying the following:

- ongoing support systems
- ongoing strategies
- outlook for the next year's practice.

Group exercise: closure   *30–90 min*

For the last gathering of the group, it is good to look back on the experience, look forward, and look inward at the group. This session should be a time to review and acknowledge all the hard work that went into the exercises. This last session should be personalised by the group in a way that participants feel most appropriate to their experience.

Conclusion

The intention of this chapter has been to raise awareness of key skills underlying reflective practice, and to encourage and support professional practitioners in assessing and developing these skills, through undertaking a series of structured exercises. It is evident that these skills are not separate elements, but are inter-related parts of a whole reflective process. While breaking down the process of reflective practice into constituent parts may be helpful as a strategy for learning and teaching, the challenge comes with combining and integrating the different elements. It is important to remember that genuine reflective practice can only be developed by becoming immersed in actually doing it. This is essential for developing an approach to professional practice, or a way of thinking, whereby one constantly reviews practice in order to learn and to improve standards of care.

Acknowledgements

This chapter draws significantly on the following unpublished work:

Atkins, S. & Murphy, K. (1993) *Developing skills for profiling learning.* An unpublished open learning package. Oxford Brookes University, Oxford.
Mackin, J. (1997) *Reflections in the mirror of experience: Understanding the ethical dilemmas of nursing practice.* Unpublished doctoral dissertation and open learning package. Teachers College, Columbia University, New York.

My sincere thanks go to Kathy Murphy and Janet Mackin for their contributions.

References

Argyris, C., Putman, R. & Smith, D.M. (1985) *Action Science.* Jossey Bass, San Francisco.
Atkins, S. & Murphy, K. (1993) Reflection: a review of the literature. *Journal of Advanced Nursing,* **18**, 1188–92.

Bloom, B.S., Englehart, M.D., Furst, E.J., Hill, W.H. & Krathwohl, D.R. (1956) *Taxonomy of Educational Objectives, Handbook 1: Cognitive Domain.* Longman, London.

Bolton, G. (2001) *Reflective practice: Writing and professional development.* Paul Chapman Publishing, London.

Boud, D., Keogh, R. & Walker, D. (1985) Promoting reflection in learning: a model. In: *Reflection: Turning Experience into Learning,* (eds D. Boud, R. Keogh & D. Walker), pp. 18–39. Kogan Page, London.

Boyd, E.M. & Fales, A.W. (1983) Reflective learning: key to learning from experience. *Journal of Humanistic Psychology,* **23**(2), 99–117.

Brockbank, A. & McGill, I. (1998) *Facilitating Reflective Learning in Higher Education.* Society for Research into Higher Education (SRHE)/Open University Press, Buckingham.

Brookfield, S.D. (1987) *Developing Critical Thinkers: Challenging Adults to Explore Alternative Ways of Thinking and Acting.* Open University Press, Milton Keynes.

Broome, A. (1998) *Managing Change,* 2nd edn. Macmillan, London.

Burnard, P. (1992) *Know Yourself! Self-awareness Activities for Nurses.* Scutari Press, Harrow.

Burnes, B. (2000) *Managing Change: A Strategic Approach to Organisational Dynamics,* 3rd edn. Pitman, London.

Burrows, D.E. (1995) The nurse teacher's role in the promotion of reflective practice. *Nurse Education Today,* **15**, 346–50.

Burton, A.J. (2000) Reflection: nursing's practice and education panacea? *Journal of Advanced Nursing,* **31**(5), 1009–17.

Carper, B.A. (1978) Fundamental Patterns of Knowing in Nursing. *Advances in Nursing Science-Practice Orientated Theory,* **1** (1), 13–23.

Carper, B. (1992) Philosophical inquiry in nursing: an application. In: *Philosophical Inquiry in Nursing* (eds J.F. Kiruchi & H. Simmons) Sage, Newbury Park.

Clarke, B., James, C. & Kelly, J. (1996) Reflective practice: reviewing the issues and refocusing the debate. *International Journal of Nursing Studies,* **33**, 171–80.

Daly, W.H. (1998) Critical thinking as an outcome of nursing education. What is it? Why is it important to nursing practice? *Journal of Advanced Nursing,* **28** (2), 323–31.

Duke, S. & Appleton, J. (2000) The use of reflection in a palliative care programme: a quantitative study of the development of reflective skills over an academic year. *Journal of Advanced Nursing,* **32** (6), 1557–68.

Durgahee, T. (1996) Promoting reflection in post-graduate nursing: a theoretical model. *Nurse Education Today,* **16**, 419–26.

Durgahee, T. (1998) Facilitating reflection: from a sage on stage to a guide on the side. *Nurse Education Today,* **18**, 419–26.

Fisher, A. (1995) *Infusing Critical Thinking into the College Curriculum.* Centre for Research in Critical Thinking, University of East Anglia, Norwich.

Gibbs, G. (1988) *Learning by Doing: A guide to teaching and learning methods.* Further Education Unit, Oxford Polytechnic, Oxford.

Glaze, J.E. (2001) Reflection as a transforming process: student advanced nurse practitioners' experiences of developing reflective skills as part of an MSc programme. *Journal of Advanced Nursing,* **34** (5), 639–47.

Greenwood, J. (1998) The role of reflection in single and double loop learning. *Journal of Advanced Nursing,* **27**, 1048–53.

Higgs, J. & Titchen, A. (2000) Knowledge and reasoning. In: *Clinical Reasoning in the Health Professions,* 2nd edn (eds J. Higgs & M. Jones). Butterworth Heinemann, Oxford.

Jasper, M.A. (1999) Nurses' perceptions of the value of written reflection. *Nurse Education Today,* **19**, 452–63.

Johns, C.C. (1995) Framing learning through reflection with Carper's fundamental ways of knowing. *Journal of Advanced Nursing* **22**, 226–34.

Johns C.C. (1996) Using a reflective model of nursing and guided reflection. *Nursing Standard*, **11** (2), 34–8.

Johns, C. (2000) *Becoming a Reflective Practitioner*. Blackwell Science, Oxford.

Kim, H. S. (1999) Critical reflective inquiry for knowledge development in nursing practice. *Journal of Advanced Nursing*, **29** (5), 1205–12.

Light, G. & Cox, R. (2001) *Learning & Teaching in Higher Education: The Reflective Professional*. Paul Chapman Publishing, London.

McGill, I. & Beaty, L. (2001) *Action Learning: a guide for professional, management & educational development*, 2nd edn. Kogan Page, London.

Mezirow, J. (1981) A critical theory of adult learning and education. *Adult Education*, **32** (1), 3–24.

Page, S. & Meerabeau, L. (2000) Achieving change through reflective practice: closing the loop. *Nurse Education Today*, **20**, 365–72.

Paget, T. (2001) Reflective practice and clinical outcomes: practitioners' views on how reflective practice has influenced their clinical practice. *Journal of Clinical Nursing*, **10**, 204–14.

Paterson, B.L. (1995) Developing and maintaining reflection in clinical journals. *Nurse Education Today*, **15**, 211–20.

Polanyi, M. (1958) *Personal Knowledge: Towards a Post-Critical Philosophy*. Routledge & Kegan Paul, London.

Scanlan, J.M. & Chernomas, W.M. (1997) Developing the reflective teacher. *Journal of Advanced Nursing*, **25**, 1138–43.

Schön, D. (1991) *The Reflective Practitioner*, 2nd edn. Jossey Bass, San Francisco.

Siegal, H. (1988) *Educating Reason: Rationality, Critical Thinking and Education*. Routledge, London.

Styles, M.M. & Moccia, P. (eds) (1993) *On Nursing: A Literary Celebration*. National League for Nursing, New York.

Wong, F., Loke, A., Wong, M., Tse, H., Kan, E. & Kember, D. (1997) An action research study into the development of nurses as reflective practitioners. *Journal of Nursing Education*, **36** (10), 476–81.

Chapter 3
Assessing and Evaluating Reflection

Sue Schutz, Carrie Angove and Pam Sharp

Introduction

Sumison and Fleet (1996) state that little is known about how reflection and reflective practice are best promoted or measured. Although this may seem to be a rather negative point on which to begin this chapter, there really is little empirical evidence on which to base the points that we wish to make. The body of evidence on reflection has continued to grow since the last edition of this book, as can be seen in Chapter 1; however, the assessment and evaluation of reflection remains a contentious area. Notwithstanding this, the aims of this chapter are to:

- Define the meanings of assessment and evaluation of reflection in nursing and explore the practical and theoretical issues that this raises.
- Outline and debate the existing evidence base for the assessment and evaluation of reflection.
- Give some practical exemplars and tools for the assessment and evaluation of reflection.

The very fact that the process of reflection lacks definition is an obstacle in its promotion (Newell 1994), and this poses difficulties for the assessment and evaluation of reflection. The current emphasis in health care on evidence-based practice makes this lack of evidence a pertinent issue and many authors raise this (Greenwood 1993; Burnard 1995; Johns 1995; Wallace 1996; Mallik 1998; Paget 2001).

Definitions

Discussion about definitions of assessment and evaluation of reflection begin with the debate about what reflection actually is. Chris Bulman offers some help with this in Chapter 1 and emphasises the issues worth considering when searching for a definition of reflection. Cotton (2001) and Watson (2002) also note the problem of definition and Hargreaves (1997, p.227) sums this up in this way:

> 'the assessment of good reflective practice is difficult as we are not certain what it is that we are looking for.'

It is no surprise therefore that there is no widely accepted method of assessing reflection (Stewart & Richardson 2000). At this stage it is important to be clear about the terminology that we are using. The terms assessment and evaluation are sometimes used interchangeably and, in the context in which we are going to explore these activities, this would be confusing. Burnard (1988) distinguishes between the two in the context of reflective journal writing. He states that to assess is to:

> 'identify a particular state at a particular time, usually with a view to taking action to change or modify that state.' (p.105)

and that evaluation is to:

> 'place a value on a course of action, to identify the success or otherwise of a course of action' (p.105)

With this in mind, we can see that to assess reflection and to evaluate it are two rather different activities. Indeed they have different aims, processes and structures. The assessment of reflection may involve different people to those involved in evaluation and the timing is likely to vary. Commonly, when the assessment of reflection is raised, this refers to the ways in which students undertaking discrete educational activities are tested in their ability to reflect on their own and others' practice. It embraces the process of reflection, the possession of the skills for reflection and the outcomes of reflection in terms of practice change. An example of this would be the assessment of an adult nursing student's written reflection on her own practice, which is contained within a learning contract. The assessor uses specific tools in order to make a judgement about the level of reflection achieved.

When the evaluation of reflection is raised, we will be referring to activities that aim to uncover the value of reflection in the educational curriculum, or in nursing practice. An example of this might be the annual review of a nursing degree programme by the higher education organisation, which asks the programme team to undertake a review of the use of reflection in that course.

The assessment of reflection

Many aspects of nursing practice and education have an impact on the assessment of reflection; in particular, the setting in which students are in practice. This may be within an institution or in the community, but it is always within the broad framework of health care. The complexities of the health service are familiar to us all, but it is worth spending some time exploring what it is about a health care setting that has an impact on reflective practice and its assessment.

The health care context

The health care context encompasses the health care organisation as a whole and the quality of leadership and management within that organisation. Constant change within health care is a fact of life and it is generally recognised that this perpetual motion is due to the impact of political, technological and sociological drivers. In nursing, the contextual component of practice is paramount and reflection can play a key part in helping the student to connect with the realities of practice. Students need to be equipped with the necessary skills that will help them learn from what they see and experience; the influence of the context can be very powerful. Staff in practice who are supervising students in reflective practice are also affected by these changes. The availability of quality, motivated mentors for students may be compromised and learning opportunities thus impinged upon. This is a common topic of feedback from staff in placement areas.

At Oxford Brookes University, factors such as these have contributed to the continual review and development of programmes to prepare nurses and other health care professionals for first level and advanced practice. In particular, it has led to the development of changes in relation to the assessment of reflection through academic work and the use of innovative tools such as portfolios to map student development. In the first edition of this book, Sarah Burns described how pre-registration students at Oxford Brookes used learning contracts to identify objectives and to write reflective accounts of how these were achieved. This demanded some considerable involvement from mentors in placement areas, who were asked to read these accounts and validate achievement of competence. As a consequence of the increased pressures that nurses in the health service were facing, this became a time-consuming and cumbersome task. Difficulties arose in sustaining this high mentor involvement in the current climate and led to the search for new tools for assessing both competence and reflection. The preliminary changes were described in the second edition of this book. Later in this chapter, we will outline the latest developments at Oxford Brookes. Contextual pressures continue to have an impact on the processes put into place.

The educational setting

The problem of adequate student support in practice is an area of increasing concern and is high on political, educational and practice agendas. Several key national publications have influenced, and continue to influence, the reprioritisation of practice education. The document *Fitness for Practice* (Peach 1999), demands more practical experience for students, and *Making a Difference* (DoH 1999), specifically focuses on strengthening education, asserting that the quality of practice education should be improved. Nurse education has faced many challenges in recent years and the use of standards and frameworks through the Quality Assurance Agency has contributed towards standardisation. The key factors in the educational world that have impacted on the context of reflective practice cross the boundaries of, and make links with, those outlined as organisational issues above. They include:

- A recruitment crisis in nursing which has changed (through the measures taken to counteract it) the diversity of the nursing profession in this country
- An emphasis on the education of students who are 'fit for purpose'
- Changes to the pattern of placements in response to criticisms of a theory–practice gap in nursing

- A shared learning initiative to increase the time that nursing students spend learning alongside other health care students
- A higher education-led trend to reduce formal assessment loads on students
- Resource pressures leading to more cost-effective ways of preparation
- An emphasis on life-long learning and transferable skills.

The impact of such pressures on the context in which students are developing into reflective practitioners, along with a concurrent decrease in qualified staff numbers and an increase in student numbers, is resulting in a need to revisit the processes used to support and assess learning in practice.

Philosophical issues in assessing reflection

The great debate in the literature is about whether reflection should actually be assessed at all or whether it is a contradiction in terms to make judgements about what is a personal process. This goes to the heart of the role that reflection plays in the development of the skills needed for competence. If reflection is a key skill in achieving the learning outcomes of particular courses and is acknowledged to have a positive impact on care, then it must be assessed. The literature describes the assessment of reflection in both summative (for example Dearmun 1997) and formative (as in Getliffe 1996) ways; the tensions are about both assessment of reflection per se and about the tools used if assessment is to be made.

Rich and Parker (1995) discuss the potential for what they call psychological burn when adding assessment to the (possibly painful) process of reflection. This suggests that there may be actual or potential harm in attempting to make judgements about students' abilities to reflect and adds an imperative to the debate about whether it is done at all, and if it is, how to do it safely. Indeed Cotton (2001) goes further in likening reflection to the confessional, where someone else knows one's innermost thoughts, and where one may be judged by that other. Previously, Beveridge (1997) raised concerns about the assessment of reflection hindering the spontaneity of the moment and, as use of a confessional is unlikely to be spontaneous and due preparation made, it would seem that the position of both these authors is not valid.

While these concerns are worthy of consideration, the fact remains that nurses (and other professionals) are attempting to recognise and value professional knowledge using concepts such as reflection because they recognise the problem of the theory–practice gap and are struggling to do something about it. If nurse education does not work at ways to assess and evaluate reflection successfully, propositional knowledge will continue to dominate as the only legitimate form of knowledge in higher education. The views outlined above hint at paternalism and fail to recognise that good facilitation can help people to stay in charge of what they reveal in their reflection. Teachers of nursing are capable of preparing nurses for and supporting them through, the difficulties and pitfalls of reflection. In Chapter 7 comments from teachers and students actually involved in reflective teaching and learning provide interesting reading to this end.

Students asked to write reflectively for assessment are not usually writing spontaneously; they are able to make use of verbal, more immediate reflection with colleagues and mentors at the time and then write at a later date. Bolton (2001) cites Boud (1998) to add strength to the argument that assessment hinders 'raw reflection', but in fact what is wanted for assessment is not this 'knee jerk' reaction to an experience, but a considered and thoughtful reflection on an incident.

The work undertaken by Ashford *et al.* (1998) found that students were more free to 'take risks' (p.14) in reflection when no formal assessment is taking place. This would suggest that a more meaningful level of reflection might be possible where no judgement is going to be made. When reflection is used formally in courses to develop practice, however, some type of assessment needs to be made in order to best utilise and to map that progress; it is difficult to see how this can be omitted. In Chapter 5 Melanie Jasper discusses the use of reflective journals and highlights the fact that not all of what is written in a reflective journal or diary may be used for formal assessment purposes. Therefore, the structure of the assessment of reflection needs to be formulated in such a way that there is opportunity for students to have both a private and a public 'version' of their reflective thoughts.

It should not, however, be assumed that the assessment of reflection in students is a kind of 'necessary evil'; Paget (2001) found that impact on practice seemed to be enhanced by summative assessment, possibly because it is a motivator to effective reflection. Another benefit of assessment may be that it instigates further research into the experience of being reflective (King 2002); this would be very welcome. Later in this chapter, we will discuss the experiences of students, mentors and lecturers in the assessment of reflection.

One of the key questions that arises here is that of clarity about what is actually being assessed; both Goodman (1984) and Mezirow (1981) assert that there are levels of reflection (see Chapter 9 for more details of their work) and therefore, without formal assessment, the level (or depth) to which an individual student is able to reflect on practice cannot be known.

It is important that educators and practitioners are clear about the outcomes of the effort put into reflective practice. Clearly, it is a time-consuming activity and one that carries with it an element of risk to those involved. There is an emphasis in both arenas on the recognition of accountability, particularly in the light of the clinical governance imperative. This strategy embraces lifelong learning as does *A First Class Service* (NHS Executive 1998), and Ghaye and Lillyman (2000) note how reflection has a part to play in this. These authors also assert that reflection must have a tangible outcome and this is difficult to measure without some form of assessment of students on formal courses.

This brings us to the second issue, which is how reflection might be best assessed. We have noted earlier that the notion of 'private' and 'public' versions of reflective writing might be a possible answer; Hannigan (2001) sees assessment of reflection as one part of a comprehensive assessment strategy and that it is how it is done that is key. The same author advocates attention to the preparation of assessors and to the support of students and staff during the process.

In summary, we would say that where reflection is a key part of the curriculum, it needs to be assessed formally. However, the strategy used to achieve this must include both summative and formative elements, and be framed by a support system for students and assessors.

Problems with the assessment of reflection

The problem areas associated with assessing reflection are many and varied, as might be expected. The wide interpretations of what constitutes reflection and how it is practically applied make for a minefield of difficulties. The key issues that arise are:

- lack of clarity about what constitutes reflection
- whether it is the process of reflection or its outcome that should be assessed
- whether reflection has levels and how these develop over time
- barriers to honesty caused by summative assessment
- lack of effective tools for assessment
- skills of facilitators
- political and financial pressures.

We will briefly consider each of these problem areas in turn.

Lack of clarity about what constitutes reflection

The varied interpretation of what constitutes reflection is a problem in that students need to know what is expected and assessors need to know what they are looking for. There is an overlap in the use of terms such as reflection, reflective practice, reflective learning, critical thinking and critical analysis (Daly 1998). Some of these are used interchangeably and some are aspects of others. Many of the skills needed for reflection, such as self-awareness and analysis, are common to more than one of these concepts. Some of the expected outcomes are also common – development of practice and professional development for example. Until there is greater clarity about what constitutes reflection as a discrete entity, it will remain somewhat difficult to assess. What is important is that educational teams have a clear idea of what they mean by reflection, that this is based on the best available evidence and that this is passed on to students using it.

The process of reflection or the outcome – what should be assessed?

Burton (2000) questions whether written reflective accounts accurately demonstrate learning and development or are merely 'a perfunctory exercise to comply with ... requirements' (p.105). This raises the question of what is actually being assessed, the process of reflecting or the impact that this has on the individual (Burns 1994; Mountford & Rogers 1996). There is no doubt that those students who possess good academic writing skills are at an advantage when written reflection is being assessed, and that there is a danger that students write what they think the assessor wants to hear (Mackintosh 1998; Platzer *et al.* 2000). This echoes Hannigan's (2001) call for comprehensive assessment strategies, which take account of this by adopting a variety of testing strategies. What is desirable is for students to engage fruitfully in reflective practice – not for them to jump through hoops. Therefore, it is both the process and the outcome that are being assessed – because they are both of equal importance. Being clear about the stages of the process of reflection and what the outcomes are (Mezirow 1981; James & Clarke 1994; Lowe & Kerr 1998) is central to curriculum design.

Whether reflection has levels and how these develop over time

The assessment of reflection needs to take into account the speed at which students develop these skills over time. Reflection is a complex activity and new students may have difficulty with it (Heath 1998). Indeed it is clear that some are more naturally reflective than others and many students struggle with reflective practice for a long time. Glaze (2002) found that, in the early stages of learning to reflect, a lack of insight acted as a barrier to reflective development, and assessment during these early stages needs to take this into account. In postgraduate courses and for mature students, this is sometimes not the case because these students are often more experienced and confident people and individual evaluation of where the students 'start at' may be needed. Burrows (1995) suggests that those under 25 years of age may lack the cognitive readiness and experience for reflective practice. This therefore includes many undergraduate nursing students. However, this work focuses on cognition, whereas reflection is the intermingling of 'thinking', feeling and action; perhaps studies focusing on this mix may reveal a different perspective. What is important is that an assessor looks for a rounded sense of the student's reflective ability, not simply a sum of the criteria used to assess this.

Barriers to honesty caused by summative assessment

As a highly personal exercise, it is clear that bringing personal feelings and judgements into the public domain may act as a barrier to reflection. Richardson (1995) maintains that assessment undermines effective reflection and that honesty will be compromised. In our experience this is often the case, but other forms of reflection may offer the student an opportunity to reflect more honestly and find ways of including this in assessed work without feeling exposed. The use of individual tutorials, reflective groups, action learning circles and personal diaries can all give students the chance to 'try it out' in a safe environment and, hopefully, come to terms with a level of honesty that feels comfortable and aids effective reflection.

Lack of effective tools for assessment

This is a key issue in assessing reflection and one that we have struggled with at Oxford Brookes University. Throughout this book, you will find a variety of possible approaches that can be used to aid reflection and we will not repeat these here. What we will do, however, is to highlight strategies that are particularly amenable to summative and formative assessment. We will also give an outline of the approaches used on some programmes at Oxford Brookes University and any evaluative comments that we feel are useful.

The ranges of tools available for the summative assessment of reflection include journals, learning contracts, critical incident analysis and reflective essays. For formative assessment, action learning circles, group and individual tutorials may be used. One of the problems that can arise with these methods is a lack of clarity about what is being assessed; it is important to have criteria that reflect the skills and activities necessary for effective reflection and to build in room for development over time. On post-graduate programmes, where educators are working with more experienced practitioners, problems can still arise. As Hannigan (2001) points out, these people are often experts in their area and use an embedded or tacit form of knowledge and thus can find it difficult to articulate what they do. Additionally, attending seminars on reflection does not necessarily equip practitioners to do it (Paget 2001); participation in the process is what is important.

Tools designed to assess reflection need to be flexible enough to allow students to progress at their own speed and to demonstrate their abilities to reflect in a variety of ways. Burton (2000) points out that coercion may defeat the purpose of the exercise and lead to demotivation. Anxiety, poor memory and hindsight bias (Newell 1994; Reece Jones 1995; Andrews 1996; Andrews *et al.* 1998) can all adversely affect performance, and tools to assess reflection need to allow students to perform to the best of their ability despite these barriers. For example, Burnard (1988) found that reflective diaries which are not completed regularly demonstrate problems with recall and this can devalue the whole experience.

Skills of facilitators

The role of the facilitator of reflective learning is crucial and we have spent some time and effort at Oxford Brookes University in exploring this and working with clinical colleagues to improve our own skill levels. The role of facilitator may be fulfilled by a lecturer, link lecturer, lecturer practitioner, practice teacher and/or mentor and requires very specific skills. A programme of training and on-going development for those who assess reflection is important, and this needs to be well resourced. These people need to have some experience of reflective practice and be able to offer students a balance of support and challenge. Some helpful material related specifically to facilitation skills and assessing reflection may be found in Andrews *et al.* (1998) and Durgahee (1998).

Political and financial pressures

The never-ending financial and resource pressures placed upon nurses can often be seen to impact negatively on our ability to effectively assess reflection. It is without doubt a time-consuming activity that can be relegated in a busy care environment to last on the list of priorities. This can be due to many factors, some of which are not directly related to real pressures. Fears in clinical staff about facilitating reflection can result in excuses about time pressures, and educators need to be sure that those asked to facilitate are adequately prepared and supported. Anxiety is created through the conflicting needs of patient care, students' expectations and the demands of managers and administrators. In the absence of a clear evidence base for reflective practice, it is often not afforded the time that it might be. More research is needed which could indicate the potential benefits of reflection for patient care, and for service delivery in general.

Tools for assessing reflection

A number of tools are available to assess students' reflective abilities and it is likely that an educational curriculum will utilise a range of these as each has strengths in the assessment of aspects of reflective practice. The variety of tools can be divided into verbal and written strategies and include the following:

Verbal strategies
- Reflective discussion with mentors
- Individual and group reflective tutorials.

Written strategies
- Reflective learning contract
- Critical incident analysis
- Reflective essay
- Reflective journal or diary
- Reflective case studies
- The reflective portfolio.

Each of these has its own distinct process and form; we will say a few words about each in turn, evaluating particular strengths and problem areas.

Verbal assessment strategies

Reflective discussion with mentors

The concept of reflective dialogue has been the subject of research (e.g. Phillips *et al.* 2000) and can be planned and structured or spontaneous and timely to the event discussed. Reflective discussion between mentors and students often falls into the unplanned category, and is usually timely to the event, taking place in the context of the event. We have mentioned the advantages of the former but not the impact of reflection in the setting of care. The influence of this is unknown but one would suspect that it might help or hinder the openness of the discussion, dependent upon the particular situation. Mentors may need to be sensitive to this, and the spontaneity of the discussion may be affected by the need to find a private and neutral place to reflect.

These kinds of reflective encounters may not be directly assessed, but they often feed into the assessment process. One of the mentor's responsibilities is often to validate competence in certain areas and this is likely to include reflective discussion of related events. The student will also be developing their thinking and self-awareness in the context of real-life practice and thus such reflective discussion is likely to be used in the development of assessed written work. The preparation of mentors is key to the success of this strategy, and the exploration of reflection should feature in the education of mentors. At Oxford Brookes University the work of Johns (1995) and Gibbs (1988) is introduced to mentors, and mentors are increasingly familiar with, and experienced in, reflective practice as the concept becomes part of a wider variety of educational courses. Mentors work alongside students on a day-to-day basis and are familiar with the experiences to which a student is exposed. Factors such as workload, the skills of the mentor, and the culture and characteristics of the care setting will influence both the frequency of these discussions and their quality. Their success depends heavily on the mentor's confidence in making explicit his or her own thought processes and openness to challenge and debate. Work carried out at Oxford Brookes (Schutz *et al.* 1996) showed that students perceive the relative success of a placement to depend heavily on the quality of their relationship with the mentor, and thus such qualities directly influence the level of reflective discussion. In Chapter 4, Charlotte Maddison discusses many of these points in more detail.

Individual and group tutorials

Individual and group tutorials are a regular feature of programmes for the preparation of nurses, and Oxford Brookes University is no exception. As resources become stretched, however, there has been pressure to minimise one-to-one tutorials, in favour of groups. The reflective tutorial can be used to focus on specific events in one student's life or to address more general issues in practice. Very often, a skilled facilitator can achieve both. The individual tutorial may be used to discuss areas that are problematic to a certain student and therefore not appropriate for groups, while group tutorials allow students to participate at the level at which they feel comfortable and to learn from each other. Facilitators of group tutorials need to ensure that students who are reluctant to contribute are not neglected and are able to engage as much as possible with other reflective activities in which they feel more comfortable. A good knowledge of group dynamics and well-developed skills in facilitation are very important; students need to be in a safe and comfortable environment while subjects that may be challenging are debated. Heath (1998) suggests that mixing together in a group students who are at different stages of a course (and therefore likely to be at a variety of levels of reflective ability), is of benefit.

The role of reflective tutorials in the assessment of reflection is likely to be of a formative nature, allowing students to explore and develop ideas and to gain feedback on these. Research has been reported on reflective practice groups (Ashford *et al.* 1998) and suggests that group tutorials have particular influence on students' development. In Chapter 6 Hazel Platzer draws on her own research in this area and discusses the pros and cons of group reflection in more depth. At Oxford Brookes University, we have introduced a reflective tutorial group into the curriculum, whereby students meet regularly in the group throughout the period of an undergraduate pre-registration programme. The skills needed for reflection are introduced gradually, starting with the skills of self-awareness and moving through those of description and critical analysis. This development responds to the concerns expressed by Heath (1998) about how novices can be overwhelmed by the new experience to which they are exposed. Initial feedback from students at Oxford Brookes University is positive and facilitators are establishing a support network.

Written assessment strategies

Before discussing some of the approaches that can be used to assess reflection in a written format, it is appropriate to explore some of the issues associated with this form of assessment. In general, it is acknowledged in educational circles that some students 'take to' academic writing more easily than others. This is particularly pertinent in reflective writing because the ability to express oneself clearly and concisely is a skill that is particularly important in written reflection. Wong *et al.* (1995) recognised that students' writing may not be indicative of their actual reflective abilities and, although they attempted to test this hypothesis verbally, numbers in the study were relatively small and conclusions therefore not very helpful. Reflection is a skill that does not easily lend itself to quantifiable research methods and the correlation between written and actual reflective ability remains unknown. The beauty of reflective writing is that it enables the student to relate everyday practice to theoretical learning and to enhance the reflective cycle in so doing. Being reflective must embrace both verbal and written abilities.

The reflective learning contract

The reflective learning contract has been used extensively in the past to facilitate learning directly from practice and, at Oxford Brookes University, to assess written reflection. Very often, we have found that the learning contract can be the 'public face' of a student's private reflective journal, and this has its drawbacks. Students have found that they cannot distinguish relevant from irrelevant material, find it difficult to include the aspect of reflection that they feel they should include, and become rather introspective (Schutz *et al.* 1996). Bolton (2001) proposes that formally assessed learning contracts lead to students following 'rules' of how to do it and also inappropriate levels of disclosure. She highlights the important challenge of encouraging students to draw upon their journals or diaries rather than divulging raw reflection. Students who do the latter will concentrate on the descriptive and emotional aspects of events to the detriment of the evaluative (Rolfe *et al.* 2001). The challenge for the educator is how to move students on to a higher level of reflection, and, as Fund *et al.* (2002) found, this is about moving to a more deliberate form of reflection, which Fund *et al.* term 'critical bridging' (p.491). At its most effective, students use the learning contract as a dialogue with the mentor and write in it regularly, asking the mentor for written feedback. As a format for demonstrating reflective growth, at its best the learning contract cannot be beaten for documenting practice-based reflection. At worst, it is time-consuming and cumbersome. Pressures related to resources, particularly the precious time of qualified nursing staff, have impacted negatively on the practical use of the learning contract for pre-registration undergraduate students. This, and other experiences with the use of learning contracts, as a means to the development of reflective practice at Oxford Brookes University, have led us to use this as a form of assessment of reflection complementing a variety of other approaches.

Critical incident analysis

The notion of the critical incident analysis is not new; it was used initially by pilots who analysed flying missions with the intent of improving their performance (Flannigan 1954). Since then, Smith and Russell (1991), Norman *et al.* (1992) and Perry (1997) have described the critical incident analysis as an appropriate strategy in nursing. The technique enables students to utilise a real event from practice that they can recall as having an impact on them. This may be a positive or negative impact. The event may be discrete, with a clear beginning and end, or more general with a variety of issues arising (Norman *et al.* 1992). When using this approach, we have found that it is important to give students guidance on the form that it might take. Smith and Russell (1991) provide a useful framework, which we have slightly adapted:

(1)   Give a concise description of the incident.
(2)   Outline why you chose the event and how and why it is significant to you
(3)   Identify the key issues and why they are important.
(4)   Reflect on:
- how you were involved, why and what you felt
- why you behaved the way you did and how you made your decisions
- the part that others played and why you think they behaved as they did
- what else was happening in the context at the time
- the relevant theoretical background
- what action might be indicated either now or in the future
- how you evaluate what happened in terms of what you have learned in a specific and in a general sense.

The specific benefits of such a tool are that it can have quite formalised guidelines, allowing students to relate the practical to the theoretical, and recognises the context of the situation. These factors can help the novice and also allow the more experienced reflective practitioner to create more depth in reflection.

The reflective essay

The traditional essay as an assessment form is easily recognised. Such well-developed approaches can be modified effectively to assess reflective learning. The basic structure of the essay remains the same, but students are asked to write from a more personal standpoint, usually writing in the first person. This makes the students' own involvement explicit and allows exploration of practice using a reflective framework. An example of the title for a reflective essay might be:

'Reflect on, and analyse the nurse's role in discharge planning in a multi-pro-fessional setting'

When marking a reflective essay, some of the usual 'rules' of academic writing need to be put aside. We have already mentioned that the essay would be written in the first person; also, the assessor would be looking for evidence of personal and professional growth. This may mean that students need to include personal thought and self-disclosure. The basic academic rules remain, such as structure, referencing and critique, but there are subtle differences. Grading criteria used to assess such work would need to embrace the reflective element and give due credit for it.

The reflective journal or diary

Using a reflective journal is, as Melanie Jasper points out in Chapter 5, a good starting point in reflective practice. Keeping a diary preserves regular time and space for reflection in a busy life (Wong *et al.* 1995). By writing about our practice experience, we can more readily articulate the subtleties of what we do, and this is a valuable skill. The notion of assessing students' reflective diaries, however, is a problematic one. If it is to be used, then students need to be aware of the purpose from the outset. Richardson and Maltby (1995) used Powell's framework (1989) to explore the use of assessed diaries, they found (as Powell herself did) that the majority of students found the assessment to be a barrier to use of the diary. The danger here is that students resort to keeping a personal version of their diary and write up another for assessment; this, as Jasper points out, is a reasonable line of action, but makes the aim of assessing a diary rather pointless, because the nature of the document is subtly different. One of the difficulties in assessing diaries or journals is the very individuality of these; grading criteria would be very difficult to construct and utilise unless these too are individual, as Burnard (1988) suggests; additionally, equity in marking would be a real issue. If reflective diaries are used at all for assessment purposes, it is beneficial to keep the assessment very simple. Wong *et al.* (1995) used three grades: reflector, non-reflector and critical reflector. This seems almost too simple and we would suggest that reflective practice could be more effectively assessed than this. In Oxford Brookes University, students' reflective journals are private unless the student chooses to share the content at a tutorial, group meeting or in written work; importantly this is entirely their choice. In this way, a reflective diary is an essential part of the assessment of reflection, but is not the actual vehicle for it.

Kember *et al.* (2001) suggest that students are so highly assessment-driven that to remove journals from the assessment process means that they are unlikely to be kept. In our experience it is often clear whether students use a diary, because the very act of writing a diary as the first stage in reflecting on an incident helps to sort out the relevant detail from the irrelevant. Therefore, students who keep a reflective diary and use it as a base for assessed work are likely to achieve a higher level of reflection.

Kember *et al.* (2001) advocate feedback on reflective journal entries, but this does not need to be assessed. It could be an informal arrangement between students, with a personal tutor or mentor, and still be as effective, without the burden of achieving certain criteria for assessment. Making this slightly more formal arrangement, as Kember *et al.* suggest, may be a useful approach, but may not be so very far from assessment in the students' eyes. Bolton (2001), who fears that students may feel under pressure to disclose personal information, supports this. In general, the literature is sceptical of the use of journals for assessment purposes (Wong *et al.* 1995; Scanlan & Chernomas 1997), although there are some interesting proposals in favour such as those of Burnard (1988).

Reflective case studies

Reflective case studies are a useful tool in allowing students to have a go at reflection, within a structured format. Often, an additional framework is used, such as a nursing model. An assignment utilising this approach might ask a student to:

> 'Choose one aspect of care, explore the evidence base for practice and critically analyse the nursing management for that aspect of care. Reflect on how the nursing management of the problem could be improved.'

This type of assessment enables the student to make meaningful connections between real life practice and theoretical material. It also allows a personal approach, such that students can explore their own practice, as well as that of others.

The reflective portfolio

Portfolios are a statutory requirement for nurses and, for this reason, seem to be a useful way of assessing reflection in the long term. There is considerable and growing support for the use of reflective portfolios in education and they have become a popular strategy in nursing courses. Later in the chapter we will give some detail about the use of the reflective portfolio in our courses at Oxford Brookes University, and include exemplars and tips for success in assessing reflection through the use of portfolios. Melanie Jasper also includes material on portfolios in Chapter 5.

Assessment of reflection at Oxford Brookes University

In a previous edition of this book, Davies and Sharp (2000) outlined the development of the strategy to assess reflection in pre-registration nursing students at Oxford Brookes University. In this programme, reflective learning has remained a central component. The work of Carper (1978), Benner (1984), Goodman (1984) Boud *et al.* (1985) and Schön (1987) have been an important influence on our approach to teaching and assessing reflection. The underpinning philosophy values the nurse–patient relationship, holism and self-awareness in practitioners. We have used reflective learning contracts to document and assess reflection, whereby students used the following format to reflect in a narrative style on their practice, and to demonstrate the achievement of the programme competencies.

Structure of the learning contract:

- Set objectives
- Identify resources and strategies to achieve these
- Give evidence via reflective narrative
- Validation, comment and feedback by mentor/link lecturer/lecturer practitioner.

A grading grid was used, which utilised the levels of reflection devised by Goodman (1984). Students achieved a higher grade if their reflection addressed the relationship between theory and practice, and if they incorporated wider issues such as ethics and politics. If the reflective evidence were purely descriptive and concentrated on techniques to reach a desired objective only, students would be awarded a lower grade. Thus, the presence of critical analysis of the relevant issues was crucial.

Concerns began to be raised about this process in the mid 1990s, and these included:

- The validity of the tool in distinguishing higher levels of reflective practice
- The possible mismatch between good reflective writing and good reflective practice
- The unwieldiness of the paperwork
- Mentors' workload
- The imperative for students to include evidence of competence.

A small-scale research project by Schutz *et al.* (1996) provided evidence that this was indeed how students, mentors and academic staff felt. As a response to this and to increased pressure from the local NHS Trust to reduce the workload for mentors, the assessment of competence was separated from the reflective and academic content. The mentor's role was thus focused on the achievement of competence and the facilitation of reflective learning in a placement. Reading of learning contracts and the validation of competence via this means was no longer the responsibility of the mentor. Students subsequently were issued with a competency record, which asked mentors to sign and comment briefly on the three components of competence in each area (knowledge, attitude and skill). Reflective practice was assessed by a variety of written means, but by academic staff only. We reviewed the curriculum and instituted more of a variety of reflective assessment strategies including reflective essays, critical incident analysis and case studies. Mentors were thus able to focus on coaching students through reflective practice in clinical placements. Following this, the reflective portfolio was introduced in order to give students a place to compile evidence of their reflective development. This will be discussed later.

Grading reflection

Although levels of reflection are widely covered in the literature in relation to depth or progression, the association of these levels with assessment has not been further explored. It does appear that in many of these descriptors of progression in reflection, higher level reflection embraces broader issues than just what is happening immediately around the student, to include application of theory to practice and a change in the student's perspective. Mezirow (1981) generated a seven-level descriptor of reflective progression, which, although highly theoretical, is nonetheless useful. Both Powell (1989) and Coutts-Jarman (1993) adapted these to the needs of nursing programmes. Powell's work shows how the stages develop from description/observation to evaluation/judgement. The same author concludes from her research that nurses tend to use lower levels of reflection, except when they are in autonomous roles, although there are some design limitations with this study, see Chapter 1.

Smith and Hatton (1993), cited in Johns and Freshwater (1998), describe three levels of reflection, which move from descriptive to dialogic to critical. Conversely, Richardson (1995) introduces a way of seeing reflective development as multi-faceted and not linear or hierarchical. This has some face value, considering that it is clear to us that some students have a greater potential for reflective practice than others. It allows for a more individual and inclusive approach with multiple 'entry' and 'exit' points. Unfortunately, it is a difficult conceptual model to translate into assessment criteria. However, we do try to assess students' starting points individually, and recognise that some progress more quickly and further than others.

At Oxford Brookes University, we use a generic assessment grid (see Table 3.1), in which the marking criteria embrace the elements of reflection. The grades available reflect the work of Goodman's (1984) levels of reflection. Module teams can add additional elements, specific to certain assignments. In general, there is still a great deal of research needed to develop grading criteria used for the assessment of reflection. There is scope to explore the various models of reflective levels and there is a need for some evidence of the validity of the tools we devise. Current criteria, both at Oxford and elsewhere, remain largely untested; however, there is increasing evidence on which to base developments.

Use of the reflective portfolio at Oxford Brookes University

At Oxford Brookes University, we have developed a pre-registration portfolio which students use to provide evidence of continued and developing reflective practice. This is completed annually for submission to the student's personal tutor. It contains a brief curriculum vitae and an overview, with evidence, of the student's self-assessed skills and achievements. The portfolio contains:

(1) A self-assessment undertaken prior to each placement, including goals for each new placement
(2) The competency statements for the course including sections for reflective self-assessment and the mentor's comments
(3) Mentor feedback pro-forma
(4) Reflective evidence, both written for the portfolio exclusively and assessed reflective written assignments
(5) An outline of the roles and responsibilities undertaken in each placement and any additional information with reflective comment.

Table 3.1   Oxford Brookes University Generic Marking Criteria, Level 3.

Grade	Academic and practice learning Demonstrates comprehensive linking of theory to practice appropriate to area of specialisation with an awareness of the developmental nature of knowledge, ethics and attitudes	Evidence base Demonstrates skilled use of extensive range of sources of information and their application	Intellectual skills Demonstrates an ability to problem solve using analysis, synthesis and evaluation
70% (A)	• Safe practice is evident • Theory and practice are fully integrated, showing insight, creativity and originality • Challenges assumptions through structured reflection on own and others' practice • Critical discussion of relevant cultural, ethical and professional issues • Principles of diversity and inclusion are evident throughout own practice. Analysis of potential for discrimination within the situation is incorporated	• Locates and accesses a comprehensive and extensive range of relevant sources of information • Evaluates and appraises reliability of sources of information	• Demonstrates insight and creativity in seeking solutions • Well-developed problem identification comprising assessment, planning, implementation and evaluation • Explores new approaches in order to aid knowledge development • Develops strong and relevant arguments, using a wide range of sources and draws appropriate conclusions. These conclusions demonstrate depth of independent thought and insight • Clear critical analysis of practice and literature, which is well integrated within the work.
60–69% (B+)	• Safe practice is evident • Theory and practice are clearly integrated • Challenges assumptions through reflection on own practice • Explores relevant cultural, ethical and professional issues	• Locates and accesses an extensive range of relevant sources of information • Appraises reliability of sources of information	• Demonstrates ability to assess and identify problem and some evaluation of choices for solutions • Critical analysis of literature is integrated within the work

Contd.

Table 3.1   Contd.

60–69% (B⁺) *Contd.*	• Principles of diversity and inclusion are evident throughout own practice		• Begins to develop views, ideas and approaches that may help to offer new knowledge • Critical analysis of practice and literature is integrated in the work • Conclusion demonstrates some independent thought and insight
50–59% (B)	• Safe practice is evident • Integration of theory and practice is evident • Reflects on own practice • Consideration of cultural, ethical and professional issues • Demonstrates appreciation of principles of diversity and inclusion in own practice	• Locates and accesses an adequate range of relevant sources of information • Limited appraisal of sources of information	• Begins to demonstrate critical thinking and analysis of practice and literature in a straightforward manner • Demonstrates a limited range of problem identification and problem-solving ability • Develops some arguments, using appropriate sources and draws simplistic conclusions • Logical progression of argument demonstrated within conclusion
40–49% (C)	• Safe practice is evident • Integration of theory and practice is limited • Limited reflection on practice • Limited consideration of relevant cultural, ethical or professional issues • Shows limited or no appreciation of principles of diversity and inclusion, but no evidence of active discrimination	• Locates and accesses a limited range of relevant sources of information • Very limited evidence of appraisal of sources of information	• Some attempt at problem solving evident but not well developed within the work • Refers to literature but mainly in a descriptive manner • Shows limited critical thinking • Some ability to assemble and link ideas from a limited range of sources • Some relevant conclusions drawn

Contd.

Table 3.1 Contd.

Refer/fail	• Unsafe practice may be evident • Insufficient integration of theory and practice • Insufficient reflection on practice • Insufficient consideration of relevant cultural ethical or professional issues • Explicit discrimination evident in practice or analysis of practice	• Locates and accesses an irrelevant/ insufficient range of sources of information • No evidence of appraisal of sources of information	• No evidence of problem identification or solving strategies • A purely descriptive account throughout • No analysis of literature • Literature used is from a limited range or from inappropriate sources • Lacks critical thinking • Ideas offered randomly and development or argument is weak • Some relevant conclusions drawn • Inappropriate or absent conclusion

This grid also includes criteria for writing skills, which are not shown here.

The portfolio approach was partly developed to meet professional statutory requirements, so that students get into the habit of collecting reflective evidence of their professional development. However, there was also a sense that some of the valuable reflective aspects in the nursing programme that had been lost with the demise of the pre-registration learning contract, would be regained through the development of portfolios. It is key to our philosophy that the assessment of reflection, and its contribution towards students' degree awards, remain in the programme.

Another advantage of the use of a portfolio is that it prepares students better for post-graduate study. Reflective portfolios are used in most of our post-graduate courses (and in many other academic institutions), and students who have not used this approach before can find it a challenging activity.

Issues for students and staff in the assessment of reflection

The difficulties that staff and students find in the assessment of reflection mirror the broader problems. A study by Angove (1999) explored the perspectives of academic staff in the assessment of reflection, finding that these people held equivocal views of what they were actually assessing. A major area of concern was about the correlation between good reflective writing and its translation into practice; this is echoed by other authors (for example Stewart and Richardson 2000). Also, some staff were not clear about how grading criteria related to levels of reflection and this influenced the guidance that students received. There are a number of issues here that may have a negative impact on the reliability of an assessment tool; and it is clear that agreed values, consistent support and feedback, and adequate preparation of staff assessing reflection are important. These issues are congruent with the findings of Stewart and Richardson (2000), who explored the experiences of occupational therapy and physiotherapy students. In this study both staff and students felt reservations about the assessment of reflection and, again, levels of support for students varied. Following their findings, Stewart and Richardson propose more of a focus on the process of reflection, rather than the outcomes. This gives some support to the use of levels of reflection and to the use of self-assessment (such as in our strategy at Oxford Brookes University).

Dealing with the problems inherent in the assessment of a difficult-to-define activity requires us to consider more creatively how we can support students and staff in the process. In Chapter 7 Chris Bulman presents the teaching and learning experiences of staff and students using reflection; perhaps we should use difficult issues positively rather than attempting to overcome them.

King and Kitchener (1994) developed a model of reflective judgement from their work with college students. They suggest that the students' ability to manage their college work depends partly on the recognition that issues can be ill-defined and demand reflective judgement. In fact, we as nurses would recognise this in practice; we just need to translate the understanding into reflecting on the process of reflection! King and Kitchener's model has seven stages whereby assumptions about the nature of knowledge increase in sophistication with accompanying development of the ability to reflect on poorly structured situations. These stages are:

Pre-reflective stages
Stage one: Knowledge is absolute
Stage two: Knowledge is absolute but not always immediately available
Stage three: Knowledge is absolute in the majority of cases, but briefly uncertain in others

Quasi-reflective stages
Stage four: knowledge is uncertain, as there is always a constituent of ambiguity in evidence
Stage five: knowledge is personal, since individuals must interpret the evidence

Reflective stages
Stage six: knowledge concerning ill-structured problems is constructed by appraising others' evidence
Stage seven: knowledge of ill-structured problems is constructed from inquiry, which leads to sensible solutions based on currently available evidence.

This model has some potential for dealing with negative experiences of staff and students in the assessment of reflection. King and Kitchener (1994) suggest that first-year students could be expected to be at level three to four, while senior students could be expected to be at level four. Thus a qualifying nurse may only reach the quasi-reflective stage at entry to primary practice. Linking this to grading criteria may be useful, but more importantly the model could be used to help both assessors and students to come to terms with the ambiguities and lack of definition in what is being assessed. What assessors and teachers of reflection need to come to terms with is the fact that their role is of 'guide on the side' rather than 'sage on the stage' (Durgahee (1998). Thus teachers and assessors are facilitators rather than anything else. Facilitation is, supposedly, widely accepted in nurse education, yet it seems likely that this less than distinct role is actually what is causing the problems here. In other aspects of the curriculum in nursing, we have many more absolutes; for example we have evidence that indicates the best way to reduce pressure damage in an immobile patient, and evidence of the most effective leadership styles. But in some areas knowledge is less than clear; for example what constitutes the experience of pain, or the effects on children of early hospitalisation. The effective assessment of reflection is one of the latter problems; knowledge is not absolute – neither how to do it nor what is wanted from it – and we need to reflect on how we assess reflection. There is some evidence – both our own and others – but the problem of how to assess reflection is a difficult one. We must construct our knowledge base from inquiry and come to sensible conclusions. We suggest that the model by King and Kitchener is a useful one for assessing students but also for how we as assessors think about the problems we encounter in assessing reflection.

Evaluating the assessment of reflection

As reflection becomes integrated within nurse education, it is increasingly important to demonstrate the benefits for professional practice and health care delivery. We propose that it is only through effective evaluation that this impact can be quantified. It is argued that all educational activity needs evaluation (Herbener & Watson 1992), and indeed as educators, it is a large part of our daily lives. With the growing use of reflection in both pre and post-registration programmes since the early 1990s, evaluation of this approach is well overdue. While reflection is perceived to play a key role in the development of effective practitioners of nursing, there is a lack of empirical evidence to support the assertion that engaging in reflective practice actually changes or in any way benefits patient care (Andrews *et al.* 1998). This highlights the need for evaluation strategies that focus specifically on the link between educational programmes and clinical effectiveness (Jordan 1988). Improvement in practice is clearly the major aim of using reflection in a curriculum and this is difficult to evaluate on any but an individual level.

So how can the student's development in practice as an outcome of reflective activity be measured? While reflective assessments as part of an overall assessment strategy can be quantified using grading systems such as those described above, this alone is not sufficient. We need to address the pervasive anxiety about whether good reflective writing equals good reflective practice. Writing about practice development as a result of reflection may not equate with actual practice development, as we have seen, let alone be a direct consequence of reflection. We also recognise that measuring the practice development of an individual is fraught with difficulties, as so many other variables may have an influence. As Heath (1998) points out, reflection as a concept does not anyway lend itself to the research approaches that can make such a measurement.

As a first step, it is useful to consider the potential outcomes of reflection, as this will help to inform potential evaluation criteria. Boud *et al.* (1985) suggest that the outcomes of reflection are both cognitive and affective in nature, providing a list of potential outcomes summarised into four key areas:

(1)   New perspectives on experience
(2)   Change in behaviour
(3)   Readiness for application
(4)   Commitment to action.

Reflective learning then may be evaluated by measuring the extent to which a student has a changed perspective on practice as a result of experience. This change in perspective may also lead to changes in attitudes, values and consequently, behaviour. The learner should demonstrate motivation to apply new knowledge and skills in practice. There may also be a deepening of understanding of their own learning style and needs, with a positive attitude towards further learning. The work of Boud *et al.* (1985) implies that a change in the way practitioners think and practise is a likely outcome of reflective practice.

As we have pointed out, measuring the outcomes of reflection may not be a straightforward activity. Boud *et al.* (1985) recognise that some of these outcomes are intangible and may not be easily demonstrated or observed in the practice completion of an educational programme. Thus, questions emerge about the most effective strategy for accurately measuring outcomes of reflection and therefore for evaluating its success.

While the issue of evaluating reflective learning is recognised in the literature, a limited number of studies have been conducted in this area. Strategies that can be utilised include:

- Qualitative evaluation by assessors and students
- Surveys collecting quantitative evaluation data
- Meta-analysis of data from student assessments of a reflective nature
- Qualitative and quantitative evaluation of student performance in a reflective practice setting where students are placed.

The main focus of this type of evaluation is to find the degree to which there is a change in a student's practice, demonstration of new knowledge or new skills. The key issue in terms of approach is to ask and also observe, so that what is espoused and what is actually present in practice both constitute data.

Exploration is likely to be made around the following criteria:

(1)   Development of the knowledge base
(2)   Development of new skills or the advancement of previous skills
(3)   A change in or refining of attitudes and values
(4)   Participation in reflective activities
(5)   Clinical practice development initiatives.

We recognise that this approach relies heavily on individual perceptions concerning a learner's development in practice, and that this may not usually be an effective method of evaluation. However, the discussion that has gone before in this chapter gives a clear idea of 'where we are coming from' on this. Utilising exemplars from practice to illustrate the measurement of aspects such as those above can contribute towards the veracity of findings, much as the use of participants' own words does in qualitative research. Also, as in qualitative research the perspective of consumers needs to be sought, and the staff in placements can and should be involved in evaluating the reflective components of courses (in which they have a vested interest after all). Andrews *et al.* (1998) assert that patient outcomes should be included to determine if the benefits of reflection are transmitted to patient outcomes. Without this the cycle is not complete, although this is likely to be some time coming. Durgahee (1998) goes further in suggesting that patients' perceptions of reflective practitioners should be included in evaluation of reflective practice; that would be a truly interesting study. We are aware that this sort of work demands some considerable skill of a researcher and there would need to be robust research strategies in place to achieve this. Rome was not built in a day, however, and less sophisticated areas need attention before we are ready to approach this one. The need to evaluate the success of reflective practice is closely allied to the need to evaluate how it is facilitated and assessed. There are some particular imperatives:

- The need to identify strategies which will map change in practice over time as a result of reflective practice as distinct from other variables
- How to include patients' perspectives in the evaluation
- The need for long-term studies which will elicit the effects of reflection on practitioners over time.

It is clearly then very important that where reflection is assessed, the relative merits of assessment strategies, and their levels of success, are evaluated. In the earlier parts of this chapter, we defined evaluation and assessment as being two distinct activities, but it is clearly the case that, where one is attempted, the other must be too. Using the definition cited earlier, evaluation of an assessment strategy must involve both placing a relative value on it and also measuring its success.

Conclusion

In this chapter we have debated what we mean by the terms assessment and evaluation in relation to reflection. Definitions have been put forward and the contextual issues discussed. We have highlighted some of the philosophical issues that arise when attempting to assess reflection, and offered our perspective on these. The problems associated with assessment of reflection have been indicated and some practical solutions suggested. Tools available for assessment are outlined, with a discussion of some of the practices used at Oxford Brookes University. The evaluation of reflective practice is also discussed and some research priorities offered. We would summarise by saying that we strongly believe that reflective practice is the key to effective interventions with patients and clients in nursing. Also, that reflection is therefore central to nurse education and must be treated as such. This involves making clear and unambiguous assessment of students' abilities and working at developing these over time. Evaluating the efficacy of these strategies is vital in order to instigate change and progress the art and science of reflective practice.

References

Andrews, M. (1996) Using reflection to develop clinical expertise. *British Journal of Nursing*, 5, 508–13.

Andrews, M., Gidman, J. & Humphreys, A. (1998) Reflection: does it enhance professional nursing practice? *British Journal of Nursing*, 7 (7), 413–17.

Angove, C.J. (1999) *Lecturer and lecturer practitioners' perceptions of grading students' reflection on experience in learning contracts*. Unpublished MSc thesis, University of Manchester.

Ashford, D., Blake, D., Knott, C., Platzer, H. & Snelling, J. (1998) Changing conceptions of reflective practice in social work, health and education. An institutional case study. *Journal of Interprofessional Care*, 12 (1), 7–19.

Benner, P. (1984) *From Novice to Expert: Excellence and Power in Clinical Nursing Practice*. Addison Wesley, California.

Beveridge, I. (1997) Teaching your students to think reflectively: the case for reflective journals. *Teaching in Higher Education*, 2 (1) 33–43.

Bolton, G. (2001) *Reflective Writing*. Paul Chapman Publishing, London.

Boud, D. (1998) Seminar: *Use and Misuse of Reflective Practice*. Sheffield University. (Unpublished)

Boud, D., Keogh, R. & Walker, D. (eds) (1985) *Reflection: Turning Experience into Learning*. Kogan Page Ltd, London.

Burnard, P. (1988) The journal as an assessment tool in nurse education. *Nurse Education Today*, 8, 105–107.

Burnard, P. (1995) Nurse educators' perceptions of reflection and reflective practice: A report of the descriptive study. *Journal of Advanced Nursing*, 21, 1167–74.

Burns, S. (1994) Assessing reflective learning. In: *Reflective Practice in Nursing; The Growth of the Professional Practitioner* (eds A. Palmer, S. Burns & C. Bulman). Blackwell Science, Oxford.

Burrows, D.E. (1995) The nurse teacher's role in the promotion of reflective practice. *Nurse Education Today*, 15, 346–50.

Burton, A.J. (2000) Reflection: nursing's practice and education panacea? *Journal of Advanced Nursing*, 31 (5), 1009–17.

Carper, B. (1978) Fundamental patterns of knowing in nursing. *Advances in Nursing Science*, 1 (v), 13–33.

Cotton, A.H. (2001) Private thoughts in the public sphere: Issues in reflection and reflective practice in nursing. *Journal of Advanced Nursing*, 36 (4), 512–19.

Coutts-Jarman, J. (1993) Using reflection and experience in nurse education. *British Journal of Nursing*, 2 (1), 77–80.

Daly, W. (1998) Critical thinking as an outcome of nursing education, what is it? Why is it important to nursing practice? *Journal of Advanced Nursing*, 28, 323–31.

Davies, C. & Sharp, P. (2000) The assessment and evaluation of reflection. In: *Reflective Practice in Nursing. The Growth of the Professional Practitioner*, 2nd edn, (eds S. Burns & C. Bulman). Blackwell Publishing, Oxford.

Dearmun, A.K. (1997) Using reflection to assess degree students. *Paediatric Nursing* 9 (1) 25–8.

DoH (1999) *Making a Difference*. Department of Health, London.

Durgahee, T. (1998) Facilitating reflection: From a sage on a stage to a guide on the side. *Nurse Education Today*, 18, 158–64.

Flannigan, J.C. (1954) The critical incident technique. *Psychological Bulletin*, 51, 327–58.

Fund, Z., Court, D. & Kramarski, B. (2002) Construction and application of an evaluative tool to assess reflection in teacher training courses. *Assessment and Evaluation in Higher Education*, 27(6), 485–99.

Getliffe, K.A. (1996) An examination of the use of reflection in the assessment of practice for undergraduate nursing students. *International Journal of Nursing Studies*, **33** (4), 361–74.

Ghaye, Y. & Lillyman, S. (2000) *Reflection: Principles and Practice for Health Care Professionals*. Mark Allen Publishing, London.

Gibbs, G. (1988) *Learning by Doing. A Guide to Teaching and Learning Methods*. Oxford Polytechnic, Oxford.

Glaze, J.E. (2002) Stages in coming to terms with reflection: student advanced nurse practitioners' perceptions of their reflective journeys. *Journal of Advanced Nursing*, **37** (30), 265–72.

Goodman, J. (1984) Reflection and teacher education: A case study and theoretical analysis. *Interchange*, **15** (3), 9–26.

Greenwood, J. (1993) The role of reflection in single and double loop learning. *Journal of Advanced Nursing*, **27** (5), 1048–53.

Hannigan, B. (2001) A discussion of the strengths and weaknesses of 'reflection' in nursing practice and education. *Journal of Clinical Nursing*, 10, 278–83.

Hargreaves, J. (1997) Using patients: exploring the ethical dimension of reflective practice in nurse education. *Journal of Advanced Nursing*, 25, 223–38.

Heath, H. (1998) Reflection and patterns of knowing in nursing. *Journal of Advanced Nursing*, 27, 1054–9.

Herbener, D. & Watson, J. (1992) Models for evaluating nurse education programmes. *Nursing Outlook*, **40** (1), 27–32.

James, C.R. & Clarke, B.A. (1994) Reflective practice in nursing: Issues for nurse education. *Nurse Education Today*, 14, 82–90.

Johns, C. (1995) The Value of Reflective Practice for Nursing. *Journal of Clinical Nursing*, 4, 23–30.

Johns, C. & Freshwater, D. (1998) *Transforming Nursing Through Reflective Practice*. Blackwell Science, Oxford.

Jordan, S. (1988) From classroom theory to clinical practice: Evaluating the impact of a post-registration course. *Nurse Education Today*, 18, 293–302.

Kember, D., Jones, A., Loke, A.Y., McKay, J., Sinclair, K., Tse, H., Webb, C., Wong, F.K.Y., Wong, M.W.L. & Yeung, E. (2001) Encouraging reflective writing. In: *Reflective Teaching and Learning in the Health Professions*. Blackwell Science, Oxford.

King, P.M. & Kitchener, K.S. (1994) *Developing Reflective Judgement: Understanding and Promoting Intellectual Growth and Critical Thinking in Adolescents and Adults*. Jossey Bass, San Francisco.

King, T. (2002) Development of student skills in reflective writing. *Proceedings of the 4th World Conference of the Consortium for Educational Development in Higher Education*. University of Western Australia, Perth. Available at: http://www.csd.uwa.edu.au/iced2002/publication/Terry King pdf

Lowe, P.B. & Kerr, C.M. (1998) Learning by reflection: the effect on educational outcomes. *Journal of Advanced Nursing*, 27, 1030–33.

Mackintosh, C. (1998) Reflection: A flawed strategy for the nursing profession. *Nurse Education Today*, 18, 553–7.

Mallik, M. (1998) The role of nurse educators in the development of reflective practitioners: a selective case study of the Australian and UK experience. *Nurse Education Today*, **18** (1) 52–63.

Mezirow, J. (1981) *Transformative Dimensions of Adult Learning*. Jossey-Bass, San Francisco.

Mountford, B. & Rogers, L. (1996) Using individual and group reflection in and on assessment as a tool for effective learning. *Journal of Advanced Nursing*, 24, 1127–34.

Newell, R. (1994) Reflection: Art science or pseudo-science? (Editorial). *Nurse Education Today*, 14, 79–81.

NHS Executive (1998) *A First Class Service*. NHS Executive, London.

Norman, I., Redfern S., Tomalin, D. & Oliver, S. (1992) Developing Flannigan's critical incident technique to elicit indicators of high and low quality nursing care from patients and their nurses. *Journal of Advanced Nursing*, 17, 590–600.

Paget, T. (2001) Reflective practice and clinical outcomes: Practitioners' views on how reflective practice has influenced their clinical practice. *Journal of Clinical Nursing*, 10, 204–14.

Peach, L. (1999) *Fitness for Practice*. The UKCC Commission for Nursing and Midwifery Education, London.

Perry, L. (1997) Critical incidents, crucial issues: Insights into the working lives of registered nurses. *Journal of Clinical Nursing*, 6, 131–7.

Phillips, T. Schostak, J. & Tyler, J. (2000) *Practice and Assessment in Nursing and Midwifery: Doing it for Real*. English National Board for Nursing, Midwifery and Health Visiting, Researching Professional Education Series. ENB, London.

Platzer, H., Blake, D. & Ashford, D. (2000) Barriers to learning from reflection: A study of the use of group-work with post-registration nurses. *Journal of Advanced Nursing*, 31 (5), 1001–8.

Powell, J. (1989) The reflective practitioner in nursing. *Journal of Advanced Nursing*, 14, 824–32.

Reece Jones, P. (1995) Hindsight bias in reflective practice: an empirical investigation. *Journal of Advanced Nursing*, 21 (4), 783–8.

Rich, A. & Parker, D. (1995) Reflection and critical incident analysis: Ethical and moral implications of their use within nursing and midwifery education. *Journal of Advanced Nursing*, 22, 1050–57.

Richardson, G. & Maltby, H. (1995) Reflection on practice: Enhancing student learning. *Journal of Advanced Nursing*, 22, 235–42.

Richardson, R. (1995) Humpty Dumpty: Reflection and reflective nursing practice. *Journal of Advanced Nursing*, 21, 1044–50.

Rolfe, G., Freshwater, D. & Jasper, M. (2001) *Critical Reflection for Nursing and the Helping Professions*. Palgrave, Basingstoke.

Scanlan, J.M. & Chernomas, W.M. (1997) Developing the reflective teacher. *Journal of Advanced Nursing*, 25, 1138–43.

Schön, D.A. (1987) *Educating the Reflective Practitioner*. Jossey Bass, San Francisco.

Schutz, S., Bulman, C. & Salussolia, M. (1996) The learning contract as a tool for documenting competence. *Teaching News* (Oxford Brookes University), 43, 17–18.

Smith, A. & Russell, J. (1991) Using critical incidents in nurse education. *Nurse Education Today*, 11 (4), 284–91.

Stewart, S. & Richardson, B. (2000) Reflection and its place in the curriculum: Should it be assessed? *Assessment and Evaluation in Higher Education*, 25 (4), 369–80.

Sumison, J. & Fleet, A. (1996) Reflection: Can we assess it? *Assessment and Evaluation in Higher Education*, 21 (2), 121–30.

Wallace, D. (1996) Experiential learning and critical thinking in nursing. *Nursing Standard*, 10 (31), 43–7.

Watson, S. (2002) The use of reflection in the assessment of practice. Can you mark learning contracts? *Nurse Education in Practice*, 2, 150–59.

Wong, F., Kember, D., Chung, L. & Yan, L. (1995) Assessing the level of student reflection from reflective journals. *Journal of Advanced Nursing*, 22, 48–57.

Chapter 4

Supporting Practitioners in the Process of Reflective Practice

Charlotte Maddison

Introduction

The overall aim of this chapter is to discuss how those of us who have responsibility for the support of student nurses, can facilitate reflection on practice within the clinical environment. In order to discuss this fully I will talk about how students are prepared for reflective practice by academic staff within the School of Health and Social Care at Oxford Brookes University, and also examine the role the mentor has in supporting and facilitating reflection in the mentee. To do this, I will draw upon the current published literature regarding mentorship in nursing, and my own recent research which focused on the support that mentors require. The findings of my research, in addition to published material, led me to consider the role of education and academic staff in supporting mentors and other clinical staff in reflective practice.

Why the need for reflection?

Nursing is a complex discipline and the facets of the nursing role are manifold. Some of the qualities and skills necessary to accomplish the role successfully include the ability to communicate and collaborate with other health professionals and to make effective decisions. Consequently there is recognition that nurses need a means of ensuring that the decisions made in practice are the most appropriate ones. Given the complexity of the role, and the fact that nurses are dealing with people, there is an acknowledgement that reflective practice can help nurses to make sense of their experiences, can help them in their decision-making (Jarvis 1992) and can be a catalyst to professional development.

As a nurse teacher, my primary concern is for the well-being of those who require nursing care and the contribution that student nurses make to the patient's experience. While in clinical practice, the student will be exposed to a range of situations that will generate all sorts of emotional responses. At this time, the student is required to understand the components of the clinical situation and to make sense of the emotion experienced. The former may be achieved through discussion with the mentor or other experienced clinical staff, while the latter will involve the student questioning the experience and how they felt at that time. This represents the initial stage of Gibbs' reflective cycle (Gibbs 1988).

Boud *et al.* (1985), in developing a framework for reflection, considered the process as an intellectual and affective activity involving the exploration of experience leading to new perspectives. Thus engaging in the process of reflective practice should result in change. However, without guidance the student may never move through the reflective cycle, resulting in the loss of significant learning and opportunities for change. Spouse (1998) believes that student nurses require support in relating theory to practice and that it is the mentor who is essential in helping the student to make connections between the two components of patient care. I would argue that this is also relevant in relation to reflective practice. When helping the student understand the clinical experience, the mentor can also help the student make sense of an emotional response, say a gut reaction or an uneasy feeling during a clinical encounter.

Preparing the student for reflection

During the taught component of the pre-registration nursing programme at Oxford Brookes University, reflective practice is presented to student nurses as a valuable aid to learning. Reflective practice may be a difficult skill for some students to develop, therefore preparation is extremely important. Knowles (1984) stresses that adult learners need to understand why certain knowledge is necessary in order to accept it, and as a consequence the adult learner needs to have control over the learning experience. This is no different for reflective practice and the benefits as well as the problematic issues should be made explicit from the onset. However my experience suggests that sometimes the benefits of reflection cannot be seen until one is actively engaged in the process, and that preparation, facilitation and support are important to the outcome. As a starting point the building blocks of reflection need to be established in order that it can be understood and adopted as a meaningful aid to learning. Atkins and Murphy (1993) noted that the skills for reflection were not clearly identified and considered this to be an important omission in our understanding of reflection. Following their review of the literature they presented self-awareness, description, critical analysis, synthesis and evaluation as fundamental to the process of reflection. Take a look at Sue Atkins' chapter in this book for more on skills for reflection (Chapter 2).

It is important to acknowledge that, despite a lack of the recognised skill base, practitioners can actively engage in the process of reflection. However, if one considers the actions required within each skill it seems more likely that practitioners may not be *fully* reflective. Self-awareness involves the practitioner knowing oneself and being exposed to self-examination. This should result in assumptions and beliefs being acknowledged and put to one side; Rungadiapachy (1999) considers self-awareness to be a prerequisite for all health professionals. However, Johns (1998, p.17) acknowledges that this can be difficult when 'practice norms are deeply embodied and not so easily shrugged aside'. This suggests that self-awareness should involve not only an examination of an individual nurse's beliefs and values, regarding practice, but also the culture of the clinical environment in which the nurse practises. Critical analysis involves investigation of a subject to discover underlying components, or principles, and synthesis involves rebuilding from the separate elements to reach a conclusion and to develop new knowledge or perspectives. Both critical analysis and synthesis are skills necessary for academic study, which may well imply that academic exposure is an important part of developing as a reflective practitioner; however, as yet there is little research evidence to corroborate this. If we acknowledge that self-awareness may be difficult to achieve and that not all practitioners have had exposure to higher education, it is probably right to suppose that practitioners attempting to engage in reflection may struggle.

At Oxford Brookes University the skills of reflection are introduced to pre-registration adult field students during personal and group tutorials between students and academic staff, utilising the activities presented by Sue Atkins. This allows students to recognise and begin to develop what we see as fundamental building blocks of reflective practice. Students are then more confident when reflecting upon experiences in clinical practice and are able to move beyond the experience and make sense of their thinking, feelings and action.

My experience suggests that providing students with the opportunity to 'reflect-on-action' (Schön, 1983) can be extremely useful and can help the student to manage similar situations. However, it may be difficult for academic staff who do not have a clinical role to fully support the student to reflect upon a clinical situation. There is much learning to be gained by 'reflection-on-action' while in the clinical environment and the mentor and other nursing staff, who understand the context of the situation at that time, can facilitate greater depths of insight into practice. For example, a student nurse can reflect upon the experience of changing a wound dressing with either a lecturer, during a group tutorial, or with the mentor who supervised the student during the procedure. Although both approaches will hopefully be of benefit, reflection with the mentor can provide greater insights into the actual experience and the mentor can add perspectives gained from being part of the experience.

The idea that student nurses can engage in and benefit from reflective practice is not fully supported. Powell (2002) suggests that it is 'ludicrous' to expect student nurses to be reflective practitioners at all because of their lack of experience. This sort of interpretation assumes that reflection is not a developmental process and that there is only one level of reflection. However, student nurses do not enter clinical practice completely void of experience and are capable of learning from their new experiences. As an adult learner, a student's perception, thoughts and assumptions constitute a frame of reference (Mezirow 1990) that will guide her interpretation of experiences. For instance, an interaction with a nurse or other health and social care professional, prior to entering a nurse education programme, is likely to shape the student's perception of that role and this will provide a frame of reference within the learning environment. A student may have had a variety of clinical experiences as a care assistant, in which she will have generated her own theories based within practice.

Schön (1983) describes the concept of the practicum (practical activities undertaken to supplement academic studies) in which education prepares students for the problems of everyday life. For example, students may be taught the physiology of blood pressure, then introduced to the principles of blood pressure monitoring, then undertake a practicum in which they carry out blood pressure monitoring within a skills laboratory. This enables them to begin to apply knowledge to the realities of clinical practice. At Oxford Brookes University students have an opportunity to practise a range of clinical skills within the skills laboratory before entering clinical practice for the first time, which will lead to the formulation of individual theories regarding skill development. These theories can be utilised within clinical practice and will guide the student in their decision-making. Inevitably, the student will encounter new challenges relating to their new skill, such as an unrecordable blood pressure. At this stage the mentor can help the student to examine their own understanding of the situation and reflect-on-action, helping the student to make appropriate decisions and come to a new understanding of that skill. Working alongside a mentor, using the expert as a guide and role model, enables the student to assimilate the new information gained, compare and contrast the evidence within practice and make changes to their own practice accordingly. This will rely heavily on the skill of the mentor in facilitating such learning.

Skills of mentors

It may appear that I am making the assumption that mentors of student nurses, and other registered practitioners, have a commitment to reflective practice and are skilled in the process. On the contrary, I consider it important to acknowledge that this is not always the case. Driscoll and Teh (2001) assert that many practitioners who believe that they are reflective may do no more than think about what they have been doing in their practice. To reflect is 'an intentional and skilled activity requiring an ability to analyse practice actions and make judgements regarding their effectiveness' (Driscoll & Teh 2001, p.96). My own research study (Maddison 2002) aimed to explore and facilitate the support and development of mentors using action research. My particular interest was in the effectiveness of mentor preparation and the role played by the link lecturer in continued support. Interview evidence suggested that some mentors were struggling to understand the principles of the nurse education programme and the role of mentoring respective students.

Further data analysis found that mentors revealed limited time for reflection and limited skill in reflective practice; this was expressed in a number of ways. One example illustrated the view that academic staff should monitor the performance and progress of mentors. While this may relate to a variety of activities, the ability to use and facilitate reflective practice was acknowledged as needing support and guidance. A particular concern that mentors may not be skilled or experienced in 'debriefing' students following an unforeseen event was illustrated in the following statement:

'I think we need to be looking at how we actually communicate with students after the event . . . I think from the mentor supporting the student role there is a weakness.'

Johns (2000) describes debriefing as an opportunity for mutual support which is facilitated by encouraging practitioners to share their experiences and to discuss incidents which cause particular anxiety and distress. If mentors and students are to benefit from the process, then both parties need to understand and use reflective practice. I asked whether it would be useful for the link lecturer to explore ways of using reflective practice with mentors. The participant indicated that it would be useful, but that mentors need to receive feedback on their performance. Therefore, if a mentor is involved in a debriefing exercise with a student, there should be a means of auditing the interaction. It occurred to me that the mentor could seek feedback from the student either formally or informally but could also self-evaluate the experience through reflection. Strengthening the mentor's ability to review and analyse their own practice, logically should facilitate improvements in clinical practice as well as improve the mentor's ability to facilitate reflection in the student.

While the skill of reflection was acknowledged as important, it was evident that mentors lacked confidence in using it. One participant identified that mentors can monitor the quality of their performance through reflective practice by identifying strengths and weaknesses, and stated that the opportunity to share a problem and discuss how best to manage that situation would be of value to mentors. In order to help mentors develop the ability to facilitate reflective practice within students, the opportunity to join the lecturer in clinical tutorials was given and a mentor development programme was established. This comprised six sessions, lasting for an hour each, on consecutive weeks. The content reflected what the research participants identified as necessary for the support and development of mentors, and strategies for reflection were included. Unfortunately, no mentors expressed a desire to participate in clinical tutorials with students and attendance at the mentor development programme was poor, with no attendance at the session dedicated to reflection. The most likely reason for this is that clinical workload prevented attendance. It may also be that the ideas expressed by the research participants did not reflect that of all mentors within the research site. Therefore mentors may not consider reflection to be an area for further support and development.

If mentors and other registered nurses are not skilled in, or committed to, reflection, it may be problematic in two ways. In the first instance students may not be fully supported through the process of learning, and secondly the exposure to contrasting philosophies may be confusing to the student. In relation to nurse education, Ewan and White (1996) emphasise the need to ensure that practice and principles taught within the academic component of a programme are relevant to the realities of practice. Therefore it is possible that reflection is advocated within the academic component of a course and not demonstrated within clinical practice. Students must be prepared for the possibility of divergent beliefs and values in practice.

Powell (2002) believed that reflective practice should not be the only recognised method of learning within nurse education. Powell's concern addresses the fact that students will have different learning styles and this should also be recognised within mentors. If a mentor's learning style is not commensurate with the principles of reflective learning, this may impact upon the mentor's ability to support the student nurse throughout the process. However, if one considers the role of education to support mentors and other clinical staff in the facilitation of student nurses' learning, then the role of education must also be in helping mentors to develop and value the skills of reflective practice. This should ensure that their own practice can be enhanced and that student nurses are fully supported within the clinical environment.

Powell (2002) believes that there has been an imbalance within the nursing curriculum, where reflective practice is heavily based within the taught component of nurse education, and that the challenge now is to establish systems to enable 'grass roots' nurses to use it. While in Oxford we have many examples of reflective practice being used effectively, my own experience and research concurs with the view of Powell, finding that some practitioners 'switch off' when the concept of reflective practice is raised and argue that there is a lack of time for the process and a general lack of confidence in its use. What is necessary is an organisational and strategic commitment to its use in order to close the apparent gap between education and practice.

The mentor role in education

The United Kingdom Central Council for Nursing and Midwifery (UKCC) recommended in *Project 2000: A New Preparation for Practice* (UKCC 1986) that nursing preparation programmes should be delivered in higher education at diploma level. Prior to Project 2000, student nurses were part of the workforce. As a result, the assessment of the student nurse's skill development was all but circumstantial and ad hoc (Neary 2000). This was due in part to workload commitments of the students and to an educational approach which Spouse (2001) describes as being derived from models of traditional apprenticeship, where students learn from peers and through trial and error. By a process of supervision and support, the new Project 2000 students would develop the skills required to become safe and competent practitioners. The new approach would relieve the student from what Melia (1987) describes as the socialisation of student nurses into the submissive culture of the ward environment.

The move towards a continuous process of assessment in many pre-registration courses emphasised the importance of clinical staff in the development of student nurses. The changes would produce an autonomous and knowledgeable doer adopting a central role in the co-ordination and delivery of care (UKCC 1986). The emphasis on relating theory to practice and the importance of supervision and support of the 'new' student led the English National Board (ENB 1989) to recommend that all pre-registration student nurses should have a mentor to assist, befriend, guide and counsel them.

The evident difficulty associated with the introduction of the mentor role was the persistent lack of clarity and definition of mentorship (Burnard 1990; Donovan 1990; Morle 1990; Morton-Cooper & Palmer 1993; Atkins & Williams 1995; Marrow & Tatum 1995; Wilson-Barnett *et al.* 1995; Cahill 1996; Neary 1999; Andrews & Chiltern 2000), although despite the lack of clarity, Morle (1990) highlighted that it did not hinder the uptake of mentorship in nursing. Therefore, providing student nurses with support, guidance and supervision seems to be a desirable concept.

Darling (1984) identified three basic mentoring roles that would teach, guide, counsel and sponsor a novice in an organisation. The roles were: the inspirer, enabling the novice to identify a goal and the means of achieving that goal; the investor, focusing on the values and needs of the novice's goal; and the supporter, providing the student with the emotional encouragement needed to develop confidence. Likewise Neary (2000) identified three support themes attributed to the mentor role. They were: educational, involving assessment and offering feedback to students as well as facilitating the students' learning; psychological support, being a friend, advisor and motivator; and managerial, suggesting liaison with appropriate staff to achieve learning opportunities and ensuring that the learning environment is safe. Additionally, Earnshaw (1994) explored the perceptions of a group of third-year student nurses of the mentor role. The key constituent was that of supporter, concurring with the conclusions of both Darling (1984) and Neary (2000).

Despite the increased emphasis placed on relating theory to practice, Lewis (1998) suggests that conflict between the two is a common problem for students and can lead to confusion. Spouse (1998, p.259) suggests that there is 'an assumption that students know what they are looking at... and that they enter their placements skilled in procedural knowledge'. On discussion with some mentors, this expectation is confirmed with the implication that students are not prepared appropriately for clinical placements. This, Spouse argues, denies the complexity of nursing and the importance of knowledge that is generated by practitioners. Spouse (1998) describes this knowledge as 'craft knowledge' (p.260) and suggests that practitioners, or mentors, may not appreciate the role they play in developing the craft of nursing.

Corlett (2000), when examining the theory–practice gap in nursing, found that both mentors and students cited the problem, not as a lack of knowledge, but as a difficulty in applying it to practice situations. Spouse (1998) concurs with these findings and refers to the contrast in which clinical nurses often call upon knowledge derived from practice to solve everyday problems. Spouse proposes a model of situational learning, which is based on Vygotsky's (1979) socio-cultural theory of learning, whereby individual learning is a convergence of physical and cultural growth which takes place on an interpersonal and intrapsychological level. Within this framework Spouse suggests that student nurses require 'scaffolding' in clinical practice.

Scaffolding involves an experienced person guiding a student through a particular activity and is a model which, Cope *et al.* (2000) suggest, enables mentors to teach effectively. A student nurse will enter clinical practice with knowledge derived from theory, or other prior experience of clinical practice, but may have difficulty relating theory and prior knowledge to the new practice experience. The role of the mentor is to facilitate the closure of the theory–practice gap through a process of supervision and support and enable the student to understand current nursing practice. Therefore, scaffolding is a mechanism to encourage both mentors and students to reflect on practice, to draw on prior experience and develop new theoretical perspectives. This does, however, rely on mentors themselves having theoretical knowledge, the ability to match that knowledge with practice and the ability to rationalise and articulate theories of nursing which are embedded in and derived from practice.

As Corlett (2000) suggested, mentors also express difficulties in relating theory to practice. This raises the question of whether it is reasonable to presume that mentors possess the skills required to mentor effectively. Neary (1999) points out that nurse education is preparing student nurses for a role in which the key skills required for practice are those relating to clinical decision-making and professional judgement. Therefore the role of the link lecturer must be sensitive and responsive to the knowledge and skill that mentors require. Consequently there could be an argument that registered nurses require 'scaffolding' through the process of becoming a mentor, and that the role of mentor education is to facilitate this.

It has been suggested that reflection may be a means of uniting theory and practice in nursing (Clarke 1986). Therefore a reflective mentor could reconcile differences between theory and practice and enable students to elicit knowledge submerged in practice. How then can a mentor promote such reconciliation?

The reflective mentor

Reid (2000) explored the work of Daloz (1986) who expressed the view that mentors are vital in steering students through reflection. Reid also provided some useful exemplars of how the work has influenced her own practice as a mentor. Daloz's work on teaching and mentoring in education stressed the importance of the relationship between the learner and the teacher and suggested that good teachers support, challenge and provide vision (see Fig. 4.1).

Supporting the student involves activities through which the mentor or teacher can build a trusting relationship with the student. Verifying and acknowledging the student's current knowledge base and experience can help achieve this. For instance, when a first-year student begins a first clinical practice experience, the mentor can offer support by establishing the student's experience of health care. This may be as a patient or relative or as a care assistant or volunteer. The mentor can then identify the student nurse's understanding of the focus of the clinical placement. Gathering this information will not only help the mentor to plan learning experiences for the student that reflect 'where they are at' in the health care experience trajectory, but will also send the message to the student that their past experiences are of value and importance.

Challenge involves the development of a 'gap' that creates anxiety within the student. In order to relieve this anxiety, the student needs to seek out a means of closing that gap. Often a student may look to a mentor for answers to a problem. In this instance, rather than simply providing an answer, the mentor can encourage a student to seek out their own answer independently, by asking them what *they* think. The mentor will act as a guide by suggesting sources of information and can thereby facilitate the student in reflection on practice. Daloz (1986) suggests that challenge and support must be in equilibrium to be effective. Otherwise *high support* and *low challenge* may stifle the student's development; conversely *high*

High

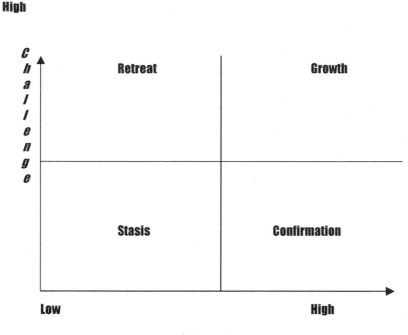

Fig. 4.1 The mutually dependent relationships in mentoring (after Daloz L.A. (1986) *Effective Teaching and Mentoring: Realising the Transformation Power of Adult Learning Experiences*, (figure on p.214), Jossey Bass, London.

challenge and *low support* will lead to a rise in the student's anxiety levels and withdrawal from the relationship, which is likely to be detrimental to the student's development.

By providing a vision Daloz (1986) implies that the student can be helped to examine and question the current state of affairs. This will promote a greater understanding and insight, which will lead to a vision of what might be possible. This involves the development of reflective skills and implicates the mentor as a role model. Observing experts in practice and constructing a wider, more comprehensive perception of a situation can lead to greater understanding of the student's own practice; indeed students seem very capable of making judgements about the quality of the practice they see and consequently coming to conclusions about how they will mould their own practice. This process of deliberation and construction of individual theories and opinions regarding a subject, is what Brookfield (2001) called critical thinking. Brookfield suggested that when one exercises critical thinking, judgements, choices and decisions are made by oneself rather than another; this is often a difficult skill for people to develop. A major component of critical thinking is the ability to challenge assumptions and to distinguish between that which is confirmed to be correct and that which is not. An assumption involves taking situations and knowledge for granted without any attempt to challenge the validity of a claim. Challenging assumptions is a major component of developing self-awareness, which, as I have previously identified, is a fundamental skill of reflection. Welsh and Swann (2002) describe the concept of 'reflective scepticism' whereby critical thinkers do not accept things at face value. Considering this and the work of Daloz (1986) and Brookfield (2001) more closely, it is evident that both reflective practice and critical thinking are inextricably linked. Brookfield suggested ten strategies for facilitating critical thinking. I consider them below in conjunction with Daloz's concept of the mentor and teacher.

Affirmation of self-worth

Brookfield stresses the need for the facilitator to respect and value the critical thinker. Engaging in critical thinking and reflective practice can result in individuals feeling exposed and vulnerable; if the facilitator does not demonstrate respect or appear to value what is being said, the individual may withdraw from the exercise. This is an important consideration, particularly in the case of adult learners. Daloz (1986) suggests that it is important to recognise anxieties in students, and to provide some structure to the relationship. When developing reflective practice, it may be necessary initially to ensure that the building blocks are in place. This can be achieved by utilising the activities described in Chapter 2, and should be a key responsibility of education. The mentor can promote a sense of self-worth by treating all the student's ideas and contributions as important and considering the student to be a valued team member.

Attentive listening

Mentors as facilitators need to empathise with individuals and understand things from their perspective. This involves active listening and the ability to read and understand non-verbal activities. Daloz suggested that listening is of immense significance to the learner. By listening attentively and encouraging the learner to speak through careful questioning, the mentor can help the student construct a map which will aid their learning journey. The mentor and nursing student in clinical practice can adopt this by actively taking an interest in the student's pathway throughout a nurse education programme, and thus assisting the student nurse to map the necessary clinical experience to be achieved during a practice placement.

Support of critical thinking efforts

Brookfield (2001) believed that facilitators need to recognise the risk of blocking an individual's attempt to think critically by questioning some of the assumptions they make. It is therefore important to provide a balance of challenge and support. Daloz (1986) asserted that close support of a learner could result in effective problem solving. Support may initially require structure, but as the student becomes more competent and confident, the mentor can partially withdraw from the relationship and enable the student to deal with more problems alone.

Reflect and mirror efforts and actions

An important aspect of developing critical thinking is the ability to view one's own assumptions from different perspectives; however, Brookfield (2001) suggests that this is often difficult for individuals. The facilitator plays an important role in enabling individuals to look at their own assumptions and this can be achieved by reflecting the individual's thoughts and actions back to them, essentially acting as a mirror to the individual, thus enabling them to see themselves from a new perspective (Schön 1983); Daloz (1986) summarised this as extending the students' self-awareness.

Motivation

Brookfield (2001) suggests that motivation is a priority for the facilitator. Only through motivation can individuals begin to realise the potential and possibilities of their ideas. However, this also requires a sense of perspective and help for individuals to recognise when a risk may not be worth taking, which corresponds with Daloz's (1986) concept of challenge and support.

Regularly evaluate progress

Engaging in critical thinking signifies a process of change in which issues are identified, explored and reflected upon, and action is taken. By providing feedback the facilitator can help the individual to judge what stage they are at and the impact of any changes. This evaluation enables learning to occur, different perspectives to be formed and actions to be altered as a result.

Create networks for support

Networks are as important to individuals engaged in critical thinking as to any individual involved in any other learning activity. Networks act as a means of support and motivation to individuals, and to facilitate critical thinking one must also facilitate the identification and development of a network. Mentors can facilitate reflection on practice and networking through clinical group tutorials with students from neighbouring placements.

Be a critical teacher

Teachers should act as a catalyst for discussion by performing a variety of roles such as advocates for non-represented perspectives, opponents of opinion, mediators and a source of information. Mentors can facilitate this during group tutorials or one-to-one encounters. This will depend on the stage of the relationship between the mentor and the student and whether there is trust between them. Clinical competence is an important attribute of the nursing mentor, as is the strength to withstand challenges to the norms of their particular practice environment.

Make people aware of how they learn critical thinking

Brookfield (2001, p.82) suggested that 'the ability to reflect consciously on one's style of learning, and to become familiar with how this might be adapted or broadened to fit changed circumstances, is a crucial element in coming to know one's critical thinking habits'. A range of questions can be used to elicit how the student approaches learning. For example, Brookfield (2001) considered it necessary to establish the approach the individual takes to seeking out new knowledge and the type of approaches taken to problem solving. Once the mentor understands the perspective the learner is working from, the mentor can then adapt to match that particular style.

Model critical thinking

This relates to the importance of having role models. By being openly reflective the mentor is likely to promote this way of thinking in the student. Good role models generally display certain characteristics, which include clarity, consistency and communicativeness. They also display specific behaviours, which allow students to adapt and try things out within their own practice. Good role models are open in that they are viewed as honest and respectful of others. Daloz (1986) believed that mentors should share themselves with others and Brookfield considered good role models to be willing to talk publicly. Mentors of student nurses need to be able to justify the actions they take in practice, but be prepared for criticism and challenge of their perspective. Finally, good role models are accessible to students; while boundaries and limitations may be established within the relationship, the mentor should not threaten or intimidate the student.

Returning to the model proposed by Daloz (1986), we can assume a mentor needs to provide an appropriate balance of support and challenge for the student. An example of this may be the experience of the theory–practice gap, in which the student may seek the guidance of the mentor to achieve closure. A challenging mentor would encourage the student to pursue closure of the theory–practice gap, while providing appropriate support or scaffolding throughout the process. An essential skill of the mentor, in enabling the student to investigate a situation, is to be able to facilitate what Daloz describes as vision, and Brookfield describes as critical thinking.

While it is acknowledged that the roles involved in the mentoring process are likely to be manifold, I think that it is fair to say that many registered nurses acting as mentors have considered themselves to be largely unprepared for the role. Wilson-Barnett *et al.* (1995) found that nursing staff often expressed difficulty understanding a nurse education programme and the expectations of them as mentors, and Duffy *et al.* (2000) and Watson (2000) found that many mentors felt unsupported by academic staff and that preparation was inadequate. Atkins and Williams (1995) emphasise the importance of formal preparation for the role, which incorporates lifelong learning and reflective practice. The challenge to education is how such skills are facilitated in practice. Clinical supervision (Butterworth *et al.*, 1998) is an approach advocated as a tool for continuing professional development and utilises reflective practice; thus it is also worthwhile to examine this within the confines of a chapter devoted to supporting practitioners in developing reflection.

Clinical supervision

Butterworth and Faugier (1992, p.12) describe clinical supervision as 'an exchange between practising professionals in the development of skills'. It is not a new concept to the fields of social work, midwifery and mental health nursing but is relatively new to those working within the adult or general nursing field. Increasing attention and interest have been given to clinical supervision since the beginning of the 1990s. Factors which have influenced this have been the changes in the organisation and delivery of care, a growing demand for a flexible work-force, the reduction of junior doctors' working hours and the introduction of *The Scope of Professional Practice* (UKCC 1992), which has led to role development in nursing and the attainment of new skills. Gillings (2000) summarised the drivers of clinical supervision as 'internal' and 'external'; internal being a response to the development of professional accountability, and external being the need to satisfy consumer expectations that care will be safe and of an acceptable minimum standard. While such significant changes were beginning to take place, it was acknowledged that a formal process of support was necessary to enable effective and appropriate change to be delivered. The desired outcome of clinical super-vision was that a practitioner would develop a different perspective on his or her work and identify alternative approaches to practice. Within the context of a changing health service, and the increased responsibility placed on nurses, Wilkins (1988) suggested that clinical supervision would protect practitioners from isolation and potential burn-out. Barton-Wright (1994) believed it to be a mechanism for developing knowledge and skill throughout a practitioner's working life.

A *Vision for the Future* (DoH 1993) and the position paper presented by Faugier and Butterworth (1994) appear to be significant catalysts for the development of clinical supervision within all areas of nursing. This coincided with the Clothier Report (DoH 1994), which emerged from the Allitt inquiry and raised concerns regarding the standard of supervision and training for nurses. This very public examination of the systems and networks of supervision within the nursing pro-fession resulted in the UKCC (1996) issuing a position paper, which upheld clinical supervision as a means to ensure the safe delivery of nursing care. Con-sequently clinical supervision is regularly identified within written NHS Trust strategies. Cynically, this may be viewed merely as a public relations exercise since evidence suggests that clinical supervision has not been widely adopted within many areas.

How, then, will clinical supervision fit within the context of reflective practice? A *Vision for the Future* stated that clinical supervision 'should be seen as a means of encouraging self-assessment and reflective skills (DoH 1993, p.15) and the UKCC (1996) indicated reflection to be key to the process of clinical supervision. Fowler and Chevannes (1998) suggested that it seems reasonable to use clinical supervision as a means of facilitating reflection, which is very much discussed but not necessarily practised within nursing. Gilbert (2001) proposes that reflection has been interpreted as a way of expressing how nurses view their actions, and corresponds with the concept of clinical supervision. However, Gilbert also challenged the use of reflective practice and clinical supervision within nursing, suggesting that the opportunities for the individual to review and modify their practice within these modes are forms of surveillance which discipline the activity of the practitioner. This 'overseeing' component of clinical supervision may be the reason why the concept is being received negatively within nursing (Goorapah, 1997).

My own interest in clinical supervision dates back to the early 1990s in my capacity as a ward manager. I was very aware that the increase in the nursing team's workload and the responsibility brought with it, created a need for a more formal approach to supporting practitioners. I then took up a position as a practice development nurse, which led me to explore the issue of clinical supervision further. I found a great deal of hostility towards the concept and that many nurses viewed it as yet another imposition on the nursing role. My attempt to address the need for clinical supervision and implement the process within both professional roles largely failed to reach fruition. It was not until some years later that I experienced a successful attempt at introducing clinical supervision within a team of nurses. My role at the time was as a team leader within a ward providing medical care and rehabilitation to older adults. I had participated in action learning, which involves the process of learning through reflection (McGill & Beatty 1995). Within action learning, action sets are formed composing a small number of group members. The aim is that individuals can learn together through reflection on their own experiences. It was at this time that I realised the potential for reflective practice to be a vehicle for clinical supervision.

Many of the widely acknowledged difficulties within the NHS and the nursing profession were experienced within the team. Shortage of staff and an increased reliance upon agency nurses, limited bed availability throughout the Trust and an increase in the medical complexity of patients, had the potential to cause anxiety among members of staff. These factors convinced me that a structured support system needed to be in place, at the very least to maintain staff morale and ensure patient safety.

Initially, I obtained support from my ward manager to establish a system of clinical supervision. Letters were then distributed to each registered nurse asking if they would be interested in listening to a short presentation on clinical supervision, with a view to adopting it as a means of support within the nursing team. All members of staff, including regular night staff, expressed an interest. The approach I took was to provide the staff with the information regarding clinical supervision and then leave the decision to participate with them. This reflects the view that it is necessary to discuss and agree the purpose of clinical supervision, as well as the process and focus of the operation (Gillings 2000). It is important to 'sell' the concept in a way that practitioners perceive it to be accessible and applicable. My own approach to selling the concept was to emphasise my belief that clinical supervision should be a method of support as opposed to a method of surveillance.

As a facilitator of clinical supervision within a practice setting, I became aware of my role as change agent. Chinn and Benne (1976) outlined three strategies for change:

(1) The empirical–rational strategy which assumes that people will adapt to change if it is demonstrated to be logical and of benefit to the organisation.
(2) The normative–re-educative strategy which recognises the cultural and social implications of change. The basic principle is collaboration, which will, with necessary education, result in ownership of the change.
(3) The power–coercive approach whereby the impetus for change comes from sources in authority, and sanctions may be used to ensure that changes occur.

It was on reflection of these strategies that I considered other possible reasons why nurses in my previous roles had not responded positively to the concept of clinical supervision. I had failed to adopt an approach that empowered individuals within the process. I was in a perceived position of authority, which may have raised suspicion that the organisation was motivated to introduce clinical supervision in order to exert further control over staff. Therefore, when attempting to introduce clinical supervision at this stage it seemed logical to adopt the normative–re-educative strategy in order to successfully facilitate it.

Ability to influence change is based on expertise and interpersonal skills (Strunk 1995). I considered that my professional experience and 'hands on' role as a team leader would provide credibility to my role as the facilitator of clinical supervision. I had a good relationship with staff and I considered that my role as team leader would provide some degree of authority and insight into organisational issues; therefore any misunderstandings regarding 'management agendas' could be explored and clarified with me.

Following the response to the initial letters, I delivered a short presentation on clinical supervision. The aim was to clarify its meaning and process and to explore reflective practice and its function within clinical supervision. The sessions also gave staff the opportunity to decide whether they wished to participate. Staff were divided into three groups each comprising 6–8 people. Group members were selected from each of the ward teams, providing a mix of grades and experience levels. The aim was to ensure that there was opportunity for open dialogue across the nursing team. During each session I discussed the ways in which clinical supervision could be delivered. Wright et al. (1997) suggested that it can be facilitated in a variety of ways and that nurses should choose which approach is more suited to them. The dyadic or one-to-one approach is described by Wilkins (1988), and involves regular one-to-one sessions with a peer or outsider as supervisor. Hawkins and Shohet (1989) discuss the concept of group supervision; it has the benefit of enabling participants to obtain greater breadth of support and perspectives of their experience through their peers.

Group supervision can be facilitated by an external supervisor or by a peer. The staff from the three groups generally agreed that the group approach would be the most appropriate, with myself as the supervisor. This is reflective of peer supervision, which Hawkins and Shohet (1989) suggest could involve rotating the facilitator role between group members. This approach can present difficulties, especially if group members lack facilitation skills. The group acknowledged this possibility but elected me as the facilitator in the first instance, with a view to rotating the responsibility once the group had become experienced in the process. As it would have proved difficult to act as a supervisor to the three groups simultaneously, I negotiated a staggered approach where group one commenced group supervision six weeks before group two, and group two commenced group supervision six weeks before group three. I anticipated that by the end of the first six weeks, group one would be in a position to adopt peer supervision.

Each supervision group was asked to negotiate their own ground rules. Each group decided on confidentiality, trust and respect of other people's viewpoints as important ground rules. As the supervisor, I later realised that I should have negotiated some ground rules with the groups. I found myself at times trying to help group members manage personal conflicts, rather than issues relating to practice. I also sensed that group members had anticipated that I would solve any interpersonal disputes by acting as a mediator in the event of team conflict.

Advocates of clinical supervision indicate the importance of reflective practice within the process; Johns (2000) discusses the concept of guided reflection in which reflection is facilitated by a guide or supervisor. Most of the group members were aware of reflection but only one 'admitted' to regularly using it as a tool for development. In order to ensure that group members were able to reflect and obtain maximum benefit from clinical supervision, I developed a reflective record form (Fig. 4.2), which was based on Gibbs' (1988) cycle of reflection. The intention was to give group members a guide, with specific questions which would facilitate reflection prior to attending a supervision session. If an incident occurred in practice, the group member could utilise a structured approach to reflect upon it and then bring the written reflection to the session.

During each session I made field notes so I could write a summary of each session for group members to retain. The information proved to be of use in the evaluation of the process. The model of clinical supervision frequently referred to and described by Butterworth and Faugier (1992) is Proctor's (1986) model, which suggests clinical supervision has three main functions: formative/educative, restorative/supportive and normative/management. Using these functions of clinical supervision as a framework, I was able to evaluate the outcome of each session. The following example brought along by a group member demonstrates this further.

'I was on a late shift. This patient had been agitated during the shift and kept asking for his named nurse. When I explained that his nurse was not on duty, he became even more agitated. He often expressed that his named nurse was the only person who could look after him properly. He kept following me about the ward and prodding me with his walking stick. I tried to reason with him, explaining that I was busy with the drug round, but he wouldn't leave me alone. I then tried to walk him back to his room, taking hold of his arm. He then started shouting at me and hitting. There were several patients sitting around who were clearly frightened. Again, I tried to reason with him but he just became more aggressive. He twisted my arm around my back. When another nurse came to help he picked up the television and threw it at her. Another patient tried to stop

REFLECTIVE PRACTICE RECORD FORM

Description:--

Feelings:--

Evaluation:--

Analysis:--

Conclusion:--

Action plan:---

Fig. 4.2   Reflective practice record form.

him so he picked up a squash bottle and hit him over the head. Eventually the on-call doctor came. We restrained the patient and the doctor sedated him. At the time it seemed like the right thing to do, but now I feel uncomfortable about it.

During the analysis stage of the reflective process the discussion identified several themes. Group members were unclear of the legal implications of restraining a patient. This prompted an action point for the group to review current guidelines and protocols pertaining to the restraint of patients. This resulted in a standard protocol being developed by the group, with the intention of ensuring that systems are in place to avoid similar situations occurring in practice. This reflected the formative/educative aspect of clinical supervision, which is concerned with the development of practice. A further theme observed was that there had been a lack of communication between the team and the patient's named nurse, both verbally and in the form of a written care plan. Clearly the named nurse was able to care for the patient in a way which ensured that the patient remained calm and free from anxiety. Difficulties arose when other team members were unable to continue that care. The agreed action point was that the named nurse should be asked to share her valuable knowledge and experience and she assisted in the development of a written care plan. The fact that the group member was able to discuss such a difficult clinical experience in a safe environment, relates to the restorative/supportive aspect of clinical supervision. The function of clinical supervision, which relates to patient protection, is the normative/management aspect of clinical supervision. By allowing open discussion and exploring policy and guidelines, clinical supervision contributed to the future safety of patients who are themselves agitated or who witness such situations. It also contributes to the future safety of health care workers, by providing a better understanding of situations that lead to aggression and of how to manage them effectively.

Conclusion

The essence of this chapter has been to suggest strategies to support practitioners in the process of reflection, with the focus on how mentors and others involved in supporting student nurses in clinical practice, can help them develop the fundamental skills of reflection. By acquiring these skills, an improved knowledge and understanding of clinical practice will hopefully become apparent. The importance of preparing student nurses for reflection has been considered, along with examples of how this is undertaken at Oxford Brookes University. The significant role of the mentor in facilitating reflection-on-action in a student nurse is also acknowledged. In order to enable a student to make connections between theory and practice, the mentor's own self-awareness and ability to engage in the process of reflection is fundamental to the support they give. To help mentors develop an increased awareness and competence in this process of learning, I have considered how strategies to develop critical thinking (Brookfield 2001) can be combined with the concept of challenge and support (Daloz 1986). Thus the ideal state for reflection-on-action is one where there is an opportunity to consider situations critically while in receipt of an equal balance of challenge and support.

The challenge of how the profile of reflective practice can be raised within clinical practice has been considered, thus the concept of clinical supervision and the relationship it has with reflection has been explored. While the potential difficulties and barriers to the implementation of clinical supervision are recognised, it must not be considered an unrealistic prospect. Therefore an example of how I implemented clinical supervision within a team of nurses, and the beneficial outcomes, is given. It is recognised that, if it is to be successful, clinical teams must take ownership of the process and make choices and decisions as to how supervision will be organised and disseminated within differing clinical environments. I believe there is a significant argument for reflection and clinical supervision to be a major component of continuing professional development, and health care providers must adopt a considerable commitment to this.

This chapter, and indeed this book, can provide guidance for practitioners in developing the skills needed to become reflective practitioners and mentors. The challenges to begin with are whether practitioners want to become actively engaged in the process of reflection, and if they do whether they are able to invest the time and energy required. Time is of particular significance in relation to clinical supervision and I encourage practitioners to seek commitment from their managers to allow time for this activity.

References

Andrews, M. & Chiltern, F. (2000) Student and mentor perceptions of mentoring effectiveness. *Nurse Education Today*, **20**, 555–62.

Atkins, S. & Murphy, K. (1993) Reflection: A review of the literature. *Journal of Advanced Nursing*, **18**, 1188–92.

Atkins, S. & Williams, A. (1995) Registered nurses' experiences of mentoring undergraduate student nurses. *Journal of Advanced Nursing*, **21**, 1006–15.

Barton-Wright, P. (1994) Clinical supervision in primary nursing. *British Journal of Nursing*, **3**(1), 24–8.

Boud, D., Keogh, R. & Walker, D. (1985) *Reflection: Turning Experience into Learning*. Kogan Page, London.

Brookfield, S.D. (2001) *Developing Critical Thinkers: Challenging Adults to Explore Alternative Ways of Thinking and Acting*, 5th edn. Open University Press, England.

Burnard, P. (1990) The student experience: adult learning and mentorship. *Nurse Education Today*, **11**, 349–54.

Butterworth, T. & Faugier, J. (1992) *Clinical Supervision and Mentoring in Nursing*. Chapman Hall, London.

Butterworth, T. Faugier, J. & Burnard, P. (1998) *Clinical Supervision and Mentorship in Nursing*, 2nd edn. Stanley Thornes, Cheltenham.

Cahill, H. (1996) A qualitative analysis of student nurses' experiences of mentorship. *Journal of Advanced Nursing*, **24**, 791–9.

Chinn, R. & Benne, R. (1976) Cited in Sheehan, J. (1990) Investigating change in a nursing context. *Journal of Advanced Nursing*, **15**, 819–24.

Clarke, M. (1986) Action and reflection: Practice and theory in nursing. *Journal of Advanced Nursing*, **11**(1), 3–11.

Cope, P. Cuthbertson, P. & Stoddart, B. (2000) Situated learning in the practice placement. *Journal of Advanced Nursing*, **31**(4), 850–56.

Corlett, J. (2000) The perceptions of nurse teachers, student nurses and preceptors of the theory-practice gap in nurse education. *Nurse Education Today*, **20**, 499–505.

Daloz, L. (1986) *Effective Teaching and Mentoring: Realizing the Transformational Power of Adult Learning Experiences*. Jossey-Bass, San Francisco.

Darling, L.A.W. (1984) What do nurses want in a mentor? *The Journal of Nursing Administration*, October, 460–64.

DoH (1993) *A Vision for the Future*. The Stationery Office, London.

DoH (1994) *The Allitt Inquiry*. (The Clothier Report). The Stationery Office, London.

Donovan, J. (1990) The concept and role of the mentor. *Nurse Education Today*, **15**, 294–8.

Driscoll, J. & Teh, B. (2001) The potential of reflective practice to develop individual orthopaedic nurse practitioners and their practice. *Journal of Orthopaedic Nursing*, **5**, 95–103.

Duffy, K. Docherty, C. Cardnuff, L. White, M. Winters, M. & Grieg, J. (2000) The nurse lecturer's role in mentoring the mentors. *Nursing Standard*, **15**(6), 35–8.

Earnshaw, G. (1994) Mentorship: the students' views'. *Nurse Education Today*, **15**, 274–9.

ENB (1989) *Preparation of Teachers, Practitioners/Teachers, mentors and supervisors in the context of project 2000*. English National Board for Nursing and Midwifery, London.

Ewan, C. & White, R. (1996), *Teaching Nursing*, 2nd edn). Chapman Hall, London.

Faugier, J. & Butterworth, T. (1994) *Clinical supervision. A position paper*. Manchester University, Manchester.

Fowler, J. & Chevannes, M. (1998) The organisation of clinical supervision within the nursing profession: a review of the literature. *Journal of Advanced Nursing*, **27**, 379–82.

Gibbs, G. (1988) *Learning by Doing: A guide to teaching and learning methods*. Further Education Unit, Oxford Polytechnic, Oxford.

Gilbert, T. (2001) Reflective practice and clinical supervision: Meticulous rituals of the confessional. *Journal of Advanced Nursing*, **36**(2), 199–205.

Gillings, B. (2000) Clinical supervision and reflective practice. In: *Reflective Practice in Nursing: The Growth of the Professional Practitioner* (eds S. Burns & C. Bulman). Blackwell Science, Oxford.

Goorapah, D. (1997) Clinical supervision. *Journal of Clinical Nursing*, **6**, 173–8.

Hawkins, P. & Shohet, R. (1989) *Supervision in the Helping Professions*. Open University Press, Buckingham.

Jarvis, P. (1992) Reflective practice and nursing. *Nurse Education Today*, **12**, 174–81.

Johns, C. (1998) Opening the doors of perception. In: *Transforming Nursing Through Reflective Practice* (eds C. Johns & D. Freshwater). Blackwell Science, Oxford.

Johns, C. (2000) *Becoming a Reflective Practitioner: A reflective and holistic approach to clinical nursing, practice development and clinical supervision*. Blackwell Science, Oxford.

Knowles, M.S (1984) *The Adult Learner: a neglected species*, 3rd edn. Gulf Publishing, Houston.

Lewis, M. (1998) An examination of the role of learning environments in the construction of nursing identity. *Nurse Education Today*, **18**, 221–5.

Maddison, C. (2002) *Facilitating the support and development of mentors and pre-registration undergraduate student nurses. An action research study*. Unpublished master's dissertation. Oxford Brookes University, Oxford.

Marrow, C. & Tatum, S. (1995) Student supervision: myth or reality? *Journal of Advanced Nursing*, **19**, 1247–55.

McGill, I. & Beatty, L. (1995) *Action Learning: A guide for professional management and educational development*, 2nd edn. Kogan Page, London.

Melia, K.M. (1987) *Learning and working: the occupational socialisation of nurses*. Tavistock, London.

Mezirow, J. (1990) *Fostering Critical Reflection in Adulthood: a Guide to Transformative and Emancipatory Learning*. Jossey-Bass, San Fransisco.

Morle, K. (1990) Mentorship – is it a case of the emperor's new clothes or a rose by any other name? *Nurse Education Today*, 10, 66–9.

Morton-Cooper, A. & Palmer, A. (1993) *Mentoring and Preceptorship: A Guide to Support Roles in Clinical Practice*. Blackwell Science, Oxford.

Neary, M. (1999) Preparing assessors for continuous assessment. *Nursing Standard*, 13(18), 41–7.

Neary, M. (2000) Responsive assessment in clinical competence: part 2. *Nursing Standard*, 15(1) 35–40.

Powell, J. (2002) Reflection and the evaluation of experience: prerequisites for therapeutic practice? In: *Nursing As Therapy* (eds R. McMahon & A. Pearson). Chapman Hall, London.

Proctor, B. (1986) Supervision: a co-operative exercise in accountability. In: *Enabling and Ensuring* (eds M. Marken & M. Payne). Leicester National Youth Bureau and Council for Education and Training in Youth and Community Work.

Reid, B. (2000) The role of the mentor to aid reflective practice. In: *Reflective Practice in Nursing: The Growth of the Professional Practitioner* (eds S. Burns & C. Bulman). Blackwell Science, Oxford.

Rungadiapachy, D. M. (1999) *Interpersonal Communication and Psychology for Health Care Professionals*. Butterworth Heinemann, Oxford.

Schön, D.A. (1983) *The Reflective Practitioner*. Temple Smith, London.

Spouse, J. (1998) Scaffolding student learning in clinical practice. *Nurse Education Today*, 18, 259–66.

Spouse, J. (2001) Bridging theory and practice in the supervisory relationship: a socio-cultural perspective. *Journal of Advanced Nursing*, 33(4), 512–22.

Strunk, B. (1995) The clinical nurse specialist as a change agent. *Clinical Nurse Specialist*, 9(3), 128–32.

UKCC (1986) *Project 2000: A new preparation for practice*. United Kingdom Central Council for Nursing, Midwifery and Health Visiting, London.

UKCC (1992) *The Scope of Professional Practice*. United Kingdom Central Council for Nursing, Midwifery and Health Visiting, London.

UKCC (1996) *Position Statement on Clinical Supervision for Nursing and Health Visiting*. United Kingdom Central Council for Nursing, Midwifery and Health Visiting, London.

Vygotsky, L. (1979) Cited in Spouse, J. (1998) Scaffolding student learning in clinical practice. *Nurse Education Today*, 18, 259–66.

Watson, S. (2000) The support that mentors receive in the clinical setting. *Nurse Education Today*, 20, 585–92.

Welsh, I. & Swann, C. (2002) *Partners in Learning: a guide to support and assessment in education*. Radcliffe Medical Press, Oxford.

Wilkins, P. (1988) Someone to watch over me. *Nursing Times*, 84(37), 33–4.

Wilson-Barnett, J., Butterworth, T., White, E., Twinn, S., Davies, S. & Riley, L. (1995) Clinical support and the project 2000 nursing student: factors influencing this process. *Journal of Advanced Nursing*, 21, 1152–8.

Wright, S. Elliot, M. & Schofield, H. (1997) A networking approach to clinical supervision. *Nursing Standard*, 11, 39–41.

Chapter 5

Using Journals and Diaries within Reflective Practice

Melanie Jasper

Introduction

Keeping a journal or diary is an activity that can be used for many different purposes. Indeed, there are numerous examples of authors documenting their experiences of living through events (e.g. Anne Frank), travel in different parts of the world (e.g. Michael Palin), or as autobiography. This chapter will concentrate on journals used as a learning strategy, in which they enable the writer to reflect on and learn from his or her experiences. This is intended as a practical chapter that provides you with tips and hints for using journal writing successfully and creatively, to recognise your learning and achieve your learning outcomes.

First, I will consider what I mean by journal writing, and explore the purposes and reasons for keeping a journal. Second, I will look at different structures for journals, and strategies for writing that may be included. Third, I will tackle the problems of getting started, and what you may want to write, providing illustrations throughout with excerpts from journals, ideas for a variety of activities, and examples of different types of writing used for different purposes within journals.

Many students will be using journals as part of course work, or to develop a learning file of evidence that they can draw from, to support portfolio claims or illustrate other forms of written work. More experienced practitioners may use journals to explore issues arising from practice that involve others, or perhaps events and incidents that have caused them to pause and think about their practice more deeply. None of these are context free, as all students and practitioners will be working in the real world of health care, which is bound by codes of professional practice and standards of care that are expected to be adhered to. I have included a section exploring ethical issues to be taken into consideration when using journal writing, especially as the journal may be used as a public document and seen by others.

What is a learning journal?

Many authors have debated the differences between the terms 'journal', 'diary' and 'log' (Holly 1988; Perkins 1996; Moon 1999a,b), but essentially I am talking about a written record of experiences. This may simply be a chronological 'diary' of events such as we would use to organise our day, or may include the activity of 'journaling' which involves reflective writing about the events and experiences that we have had (Landeen *et al.* 1992). In this chapter, I will use the term 'journal' to mean all of the types of writing that you may do that are reflective in nature and that are used to record your experiences on a continual basis. This is summarised very effectively by Holly (1988, p.78) who says:

> 'A journal is a record of happenings, thoughts and feelings about a particular aspect of life, or with a particular structure. A journal can record anything relative to the issue to which it pertains. So a reflective practice journal is like a diary of practice, but in addition includes deliberative thought and analysis related to practice.'

Degazon and Lunney (1995) suggest that journal writing as a strategy for learning encompasses the tenets of adult education, in that:

- It proceeds at the learner's own pace
- The learner selects the subject matter
- It is an independent and solitary activity
- There is freedom of expression, feelings, perceptions and frustrations without fear of exposure.

These suggest that a journal needs to be under the control of the writer, who ultimately makes the decisions over its content, who else will see it, the style in which it is written and the way in which it is used. For a journal to be used for learning, it needs to have the following characteristics:

- It is compiled on an incremental basis over a period of time
- It provides a record of events and experiences
- It is focused on identifying learning that has occurred
- It contains reflective commentaries or accounts.

(Jasper 2003)

These important characteristics are worth exploring in more detail.

The incremental basis of a journal

For a journal to document learning it needs to be built up incrementally over a period of time. This will show how the writer has grown and developed and worked their way towards achieving the learning outcomes that are expected. This is particularly so for students who need to develop to the level of professional competence within a set period of time; and who, within that time not only have to demonstrate theoretical and practical competence, but also develop the attributes of being a professional practitioner. This is often achieved through revisiting the original journal entry several times over a period, and reflecting anew on the experience. This enables the writer to document their changing perceptions of the experience as they learn more, or see things differently, with hindsight and new experiences.

However, it is also becoming increasingly common for qualified nurses to use reflective journal writing within their professional portfolios, to demonstrate their on-going competence and learning throughout their practice. In fact, Jasper (1999) in a study exploring experienced nurses' use of reflective writing within portfolios, found that the main reason why nurses write reflectively is to provide evidence of their continuing competence through their careers. As with students' journals, particular aspects of a practitioner's development can be traced from the initial stimulus, such as an incident or event, through a series of reflections dedicated to developing learning and increasing understanding, which leads to changes in perception and behaviour, and professional, personal and practice development.

Recording events and experiences

Not only is the journal an incremental record, but it needs to be written *regularly*, so that it becomes a continual record of a person's experiences, or things that have happened to them. Of course, an expectation of daily entries is something only for the very committed! However, many practitioners find that they make entries in their journals when something happens that sticks in their minds and they feel the need to explore it in some detail through reflective strategies. To do this you need to write as full a description of the event as possible. This is important because our memory of events changes over time, and the version that we would write immediately after something has happened is likely to be very different from its description three or six months later. However, it is the detail in the immediacy of something that provides the basis for our learning, as it will include not simply an objective description of what has happened, but also our subjective *experience* of that event that is crucial to enabling us to understand the event in its entirety.

On-your-own exercise: Why not test this out for yourself?   *20 min*

First of all, think back over the past few months and identify an event that has happened to you that you remember because of your emotional reactions to it. This might be something that made you very happy, gave you confidence in yourself, or represented some sort of achievement. Or, you might choose an event that made you angry, distressed or unhappy; or that left you feeling uncomfortable about the consequences. Write a description of this event in as much detail as you can remember (you might like to use one of the frameworks for reflection offered in Chapter 9 to do this, or another reflective model that you are familiar with).

It is likely that you have written a factual description of what happened, as if you are telling a story to someone else – is this true? If not, what else have you included?

Now think back to the event itself and attempt to recapture the feelings and emotions that you had at the time. Are these truly represented in the account that you have written? Can you identify the reasons for your answer?

Next time something happens to you that raises your emotional level, make a mental note to write it down as soon as possible after the event. Compare this description with the one that you made earlier and identify the differences.

These records of events and experiences build a picture of our lives as practitioners, and are fascinating as records of this in themselves. However, for journaling to be used as a tool for our learning, we need to be doing more than simply recording our experiences and initial reactions to them.

Identifying learning

It may be obvious to say that a *learning* journal needs to help the writer identify their *learning*, but this is not quite as simple as it sounds. It is relatively easy to record achievements as a list, or to write a description of an experience and conclude with identifying what has been learnt as a result of it, but doing this within a journal is likely to involve a great deal more. Firstly, you will be identifying your progress as your knowledge and skills develop over time. For instance, you may, as a student, have a book that records your skills in the practice environment, where you can see how you have progressed from a novice to being competent in the things you do. However, the entries relating to these skill acquisitions in your journal are likely to involve not simply practical competence, but also your growing awareness of the processes you are using to learn. This will include how you are learning, what you are learning, how you relate your previous knowledge to new experiences and how your knowledge is increasing as you progress through your course. This may include, for example, the ethical considerations regarding particular treatment activities that you undertake, or an awareness of the socio-economic constraints that inhibit certain groups from equal access to care, as well as the more practical elements of developing a skill and progressing to more complex nursing problems.

So while you can identify your learning through other mechanisms such as practice assessment documents, or examinations, the use of a learning journal is more likely to enable you to consider all the aspects of what happens to you. This helps you to consider your experience holistically, from different angles and outcomes, exploring differing solutions and resultant action that takes your learning from the theoretical to the practical.

Qualified practitioners may use journals to learn in a less formal or directive way, as they are not confined by course requirements. However, the processes used are very similar, in that a learning journal becomes a record of the ways in which problems are identified and solved through reflective thinking and writing processes developed over time. This process is illustrated in Box 5.1, although much of the detail has been removed from this extract in order to demonstrate the developmental process that occurred.

The nurse in Box 5.1, through revisiting the experience, changes her perceptions of the original event enabling her to learn from it in a positive way. This is unlikely to have happened had she not used journaling to facilitate her thought processes and actively explore the total experience from different points of view.

The ways in which this happens in journal writing is by the deliberate inclusion of reflective writing to help us to understand the processes of learning, and the wider issues involved.

Box 5.1   Reflections of a supervision group.

Meeting one – We began the supervision group today, which is to last for two years. Having no prior experience of formal supervision I came to this as a novice, with a few feelings of trepidation but willing to go along with it as a new way of learning. Two incidents happened that stick out in my mind.

The initial task set for the group by the facilitator was to determine the ground rules that we would all sign up to. This resulted in the first confrontational dialogue between the tutor and certain members of the group. They challenged her style in determining the ground rules by writing on the blackboard what she thought the rules should be. I was beginning to feel uncomfortable, especially as the group was so small. We compromised by agreeing on having a general discussion, but delaying writing the rules until the next meeting when we could all be present.

The second incident that was particularly powerful for me was the group exercise that the tutor engaged us in. We were rearranged to sit in a circle, eyes closed and asked to reveal our thoughts and make individual statements about how we felt. During this exercise, I could feel my anxiety rising and I desperately tried to disguise my true thoughts by delivering nondescript, unrevealing comments. I felt extremely vulnerable and annoyed at my docile acceptance of unquestioningly taking part in such an exercise. Certain members of the group again challenged the tutor as to the validity of such an exercise and abruptly ended it. It was their demonstrated experience and knowledge of such exercises that was a powerful learning event for me.

Reflection one week later – Although I was shocked at my passivity, I realised that this was being driven by my profound sense of not being in control. I felt threatened and in a dependent position, and unable to get beyond the authority of the 'teacher'.

Three weeks later – This experience keeps coming back to me and reminds me of the many times in school and nurse training where I did what I was told, despite feeling uncomfortable and not wanting to conform. I realised the other day that this is because of the central role that authority figures, rules and approval have played in my life. I was a 'good' schoolchild, and felt no need to challenge the systems and authority in what was a very didactic nurse education system. The apprenticeship model of training in the wards meant that you had to toe the line or you would get a 'bad' report. The hierarchical structure of nursing employment and grading reinforces this. So, whenever I am confronted with authority figures where I am not the one in control, I tend to do what I am told, despite feelings to the contrary. I wonder why I do this?

Two months later – We have now had two more group supervision sessions. I continue to feel extremely uncomfortable within these sessions and when I engage in discussion I remain reticent and thoughtful. Part of this is due to the conflicting messages given about the group. The way the sessions are conducted is reminiscent of personal counselling, but in a group setting. My perception of group supervision was that we would learn new ways of thinking by viewing situations from multiple perspectives. These sessions do little to encourage critical thinking about practice development per se. Despite this negativity and concern, I am able to use my increased knowledge of group dynamics and my own behaviour in considering how I supervise those within my workplace. Through this, I now appreciate diverse reactions to supervision and the need for clear aims and focus in order to achieve practice development as opposed to personal problem solving.

Arising from the first experience, I have made strong personal and professional relationships with three of the other members and these have influenced my perspective on health care and our roles as nurses within it. They have fundamentally challenged my attitudes on group behaviour and reinforced my personal responsibility within this.

Contd.

One year later – Although I still smart at the memories of the first group, the bonding that occurred as a result of our joint negative experiences has actually turned into very strong relationships. I can see now what the facilitator was aiming to do, and in some ways can sympathise with her position. I now have experiences of facilitating groups, and that first meeting is always anxiety provoking. It is very tempting to try to maintain control over the group by using exercises, but, as a result of my experiences, I never try to put the group members in this sort of position. I have learnt that for me, the skilled facilitator is one who knows exactly which questions to ask, when to speak and when not, and how to manage group dynamics. Our own group has grown beyond what could possibly have been imagined in the first few meetings – in fact, it was doubtful whether people would actually turn up again! At the end of a year we have a strong group, offering support to each other and helping them to see ways through difficulties. Perhaps a little distress is needed in these groups for trust to occur – although I am still not convinced that confrontation is the most effective way to do it. For myself, I realise now that I have grown in terms of resisting the pull of the authority figure, and I am more assertive in situations where previously I would have deferred to another person because of their status.

Reflective commentaries and accounts

The nature of reflective writing provides us with strategies for linking the experience itself with our learning. It is only by exploring our experiences in a reflective way that we will come to an understanding of the wider context of them, and just what and how we have learnt through them. In a way, reflective writing enables us to learn at a faster pace than if we were simply expecting to absorb knowledge and skills as we go through our course. This happens because we are consciously engaging in the process of writing as a learning tool in itself, and using it with the specific purpose of facilitating our learning. It is the *active* nature of reflection that enables us to acknowledge what we know, how we know it, what we do not know, and what we need to do to remedy this. The learning journal therefore provides the mechanism for not only linking theory with practice, but also for developing our own theories about practice for practice.

Purposes of keeping a learning journal

Moon (1999b) presents 18 purposes for keeping a journal (summarised in Table 5.1).

If we look at these more closely, they can be grouped together under the following four headings.

(1) Personal development – learning about oneself and one's practice

Learning journals are very personal and individual accounts of someone's journey at particular stages of their life. The learning journal will incorporate not only the bare facts of events, but also the writer's experiences of those events, which will be different from anyone else who was there at the time. Hence, through using the journal we learn about ourselves, the ways in which we react to things that happen

Table 5.1   The purposes of keeping learning journals. Adapted from Moon (1999b, p.189–93)

- To record experience
- To facilitate learning from experience
- To support understanding and the representation of the understanding
- To develop critical thinking or the development of a questioning attitude
- To encourage metacognition
- To increase active involvement in and ownership of learning
- To increase ability in reflection and thinking
- To enhance problem-solving skills
- As a means of assessment in formal education
- To enhance reflective practice
- For reasons of personal development and self-empowerment
- For therapeutic purposes or as a means of supporting behaviour change
- To enhance creativity
- To improve writing
- To improve or give 'voice'; as a means of self-expression
- To foster communication and foster reflective and creative interaction in a group
- To support planning and progress in research or a project
- As a means of communication between a learner and another

to us, and our feelings about them. In Moon's (1999b) terms, this enhances our abilities to 'give voice' to this. The act of writing itself brings more to the learning process than simply recording the events. Jasper (2003) summarises as follows the features of reflective writing in relation to personal learning:

Writing helps us to:

- Order our thoughts
- Develop our analytical skills
- Develop our critical thinking
- Develop our creativity
- Develop new understandings and knowledge
- Show us what we understand, and identify the limits of our understanding.

To these we can add Moon's criterion of problem-solving skills. These are all features that, once developed, will stay with us throughout our lives, and enable us to grow and move forward. These are often processes that we are unaware of because they are not tangible – we are unlikely to say that a particular event improved our critical thinking for instance. However, the reflective activity that occurs in journal writing charts personal learning, serving to develop the above attributes, which in turn are crucial to professional practice (Degazon & Lunney 1995).

On-your-own exercise   *5 min*

Look back at the illustration in Box 5.1. Can you identify this nurse's personal development from her writing? Use the features of reflective writing identified above to organise your answers.

(2) Professional development

Every three years, registered nurses are required to provide evidence of continuing competence and accountability for their practice. To this end, nurses are expected to compile a personal profile or portfolio that details their continuing development over the previous three years (UKCC 2001). As Jasper (1999) found, experienced nurses who use reflective writing within their portfolios did so primarily in order to provide evidence of their accountability as practitioners, in a way that was open to public scrutiny. Many of Jasper's respondents used journaling within their portfolios as a way of demonstrating their own increasing expertise and skill by providing detailed records of practice, professional and personal development. This might include, for instance, reflective activity relating to attendance at a study day, which resulted in evaluation of current practice, identification of where improvements could be made, piloting of new practices, further evaluation and readjustment, and so on. This shows that not only has an event been attended (which in itself does not indicate that anything has been learnt!) but demonstrates that the nurse understood the content, considered it in the light of her own practice, and applied it within a different context.

Journal writing is extremely useful in recording professional development because it provides not only the end result, but also, as with personal development, a record of the processes that the writer has gone through in order to achieve these.

(3) Facilitating learning

Several of Moon's purposes incorporate the notion of journaling as facilitating learning. Callister (1993) suggests that this enables the student to build a personal conceptual framework, with Haigh (2001) adding that journal writing makes the students self-conscious of the development of their learning and encourages them to recognise what is being learnt and how. Journal writing is a strategy primarily for experiential learning, i.e. the subject matter that is used arises from the writer's own experiences. It acts as a conduit between the *received* knowledge that we have (such as theoretical knowledge from external sources, or watching a practical skill) and the *applied* knowledge that results from considering the knowledge within a specific context. As Hahnemann (1986) suggests, journal writing is a process that forces students to search for connections and relationships in their learning.

(4) The development of reflective practice

Put simply, reflective practice involves completing the **experience-reflection-action** (ERA) cycle (Jasper 2003) that all models and frameworks propose. Reflective *practice* differs from simply engaging in the reflective processes because it necessarily ends in some action being taken – to 'practise' means to engage in practical activity after all. This action might be very simple, such as deciding to go and look something up in the library, or it may be on a grander scale, such as initiating changes in practice resulting in practice development. The act and processes involved in journaling help the writer frame the action that will be taken as a result of reflecting on experiences, by drawing them through the reflective processes to conclusions focused on conscious action, behaviour and choice.

Jasper's updated model of the way experienced nurses use reflective writing in portfolios is presented in Fig. 5.1, and shows the links and relationships between the concepts proposed in her earlier model (Jasper 1999). These relationships are important in journaling, because they make explicit the significance of both the *processes* involved in writing reflectively, and the *content* and *outcomes* that are its focus.

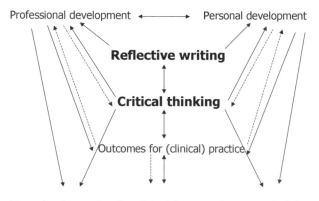

Fig 5.1   Experienced nurses' use of reflective writing in portfolios (version 2).

Styles of learning journals

There are many different types and variations of style, of journals, depending on the purpose for which they are being written, who will be having access to them and who will be contributing to them.

The solitary journal

This type of journal is totally under the control of the writer, who makes all the decisions about its content, structure, purpose, style and use. Very often, the writer is choosing to keep a journal of this sort of their own volition. However, such journals may also be used in courses where students are advised to write journals for their own development, and to draw on these later in assessed work. In the latter cases, the assessor will not be accessing the journal itself, but extracts from it will be used as evidence within the written assignments.

The 'writer-writes-reader-reads' journal

This style is most commonly found in student work, where the student is required to keep a learning journal for some purpose specified by their course tutors. Hence the student writes and the lecturer/assessor reads and may make comments in feedback. The amount of control the writer has in this style can vary a great deal. At one extreme, students are given the journal format, told what they need to write in it and given structures such as a reflective model or framework to be used and the types of reflective components required, such as learning contracts, critical incident analyses, diaries or logs and reflective reviews. An example of a journal of this sort is described by Cook (2000) who asked students to record their experiences through the course, including lectures, reading and discussions, reflect on these and make sense of them in terms of their own learning.

Another strategy is described by Marland and McSherry (1997) who asked students to spend 30 minutes at the end of each shift to review their day, to record their personal experiences and observations. These entries were then used in tutorial and group discussions to recall and analyse past events that resulted in learning of some sort.

Other students may have more choice and be able to determine these for themselves.

Journals used for other purposes, such as those used by practitioners in compiling professional portfolios, will clearly be more loosely structured than those where large numbers of students are required to complete them for assignment purposes and standardisation is required. Although the PREP regulations (standards for Post-Registration Education and Practice) (UKCC 2001) necessitate a portfolio being kept, the content of it is left up to the nurse, providing it shows that the components required to demonstrate competence have been achieved. For the purposes of audit, any journal kept by a nurse will not be considered as part of the profile that needs to be seen by a reviewer.

The dialogue journal

Drevdahl and Dorcy (2002) provide an example of a journal used as a form of communication between the student and teacher, where a dialogue style is used. They call this style 'conversing in writing' in which students are encouraged to write about their experiences, ask questions, and share thoughts that they might not want to verbalise. It keeps the teacher abreast of the student's experiences, and provides a forum through which the teacher can reply to the student's writing on an on-going basis.

Hurtig *et al.* (1989) call this style an *interactive* journal because a daily record of the student's 'ideas, feelings, actions and reactions that relate to a nursing practicum' is created, to which the teacher responds. This creates a diary that is an interaction between student and teacher. This enables teaching to be individualised, and the student to receive immediate and on-going feedback with learning deficits identified and remedied swiftly.

Another example of this is where practitioners set up dialogue journals between themselves as a way of bouncing ideas around and learning from each other's reflectivity and experiences. With the use of the internet and email, and the abundance of focused chat rooms available, this is a growing way for a journal to be used and contributed to by more than one person.

The group journal

The dialogue journal can be developed beyond two people to include teamwork and group discussion. It is particularly useful for developmental situations where group projects are undertaken or new ideas and processes are being tested. In action research situations, for instance, where all members of a team are testing new ways of working, an on-going journal that everyone has access to and in which they can record their thoughts or ideas on a daily basis is a very useful way of capturing the everyday experiences and insights that may be crucial to the success of the project.

Another way in which group journals can be used in patient settings, is for team members to record case diaries detailing different perspectives and developments in a patient's care. This is different to case notes because there is freedom for subjective feelings and experiences to be recorded and shared with other members of the team.

Clearly, there are many creative and innovative ways in which journals can be structured to meet the needs of the person writing and the type of event that is being reflected on. The choice of which approach to use is often dependent on the content of the journal itself, and it is to this that I now turn.

The content of the journal

As a private document, a journal can include whatever you want it to. There are no rules about personal reflective writing – the important thing is to use it to achieve the purpose you are using it for, and to write it in a way that you want to write it. So, where there are no rules, the scope for variety and innovation is very broad. Below I present various ways in which you might write reflectively, from the straightforward descriptive account to those which are more creative or analytical. It is worth experimenting with different styles of writing, selecting those that suit your learning style and the type of event, experience or incident that you are exploring.

Suggestions for different types of writing activities that may be used in a journal can be found in Table 5.2

Rolfe *et al.* (2001) grouped writing into analytical and creative strategies as a useful way of dividing those which may be outcome driven and those which may be more directed at exploring emotions and feelings. In using analytical strategies, we focus on using our experiences as objective data that we can analyse to identify our learning. These techniques are most likely to be used where other people are likely to read the journal. *Critical incident analyses* and using *structured frameworks for reflection*, for instance, help us to stand back from our own experiences of the event using analysis and critique to arrive at different perceptions. Many of these may take a great deal of time to complete effectively and may not be suitable for everyday use and are thus reserved for specific incidents. However, Borton's framework, which simply asks questions directed through three question stems, is an easy framework to carry in your head and use on an everyday basis. Table 5.3 shows how these stems can be used to focus your reflective writing.

Table 5.2 Reflective writing strategies.

Analytical strategies	Creative strategies
• Critical incident analyses. • Dialogical writing (creating a conversation through questions and answers). • Making a case – exploring the alternative perspectives of an issue. • Creating an on-going record. • Exploring a problem. • SWOT[1] analysis. • Using a structured reflective framework, e.g. Johns (2000), Gibbs (1988), Borton (1970). • Identifying three-a-day, e.g. three things I have learnt from this shift are. . . *or*, three tips for future practice from this experience are. . . These can be varied to ensure that the learning strategy is varied and does not become stale. • Page-a-day record of experiences. • Writing a word limited summary. • Identifying specific aspects from a situation, e.g. focusing on knowledge, or skills analysis. • Learning outcomes – using these as reflective cues to review an experience. • Identifying competencies.	• Writing the unsent letter (or email). • Writing to a nominated other person, e.g. your mother, or a close friend. • Writing as the other person. • Writing as a journalist. • Storytelling/fantasy. • Poetry. • Creating a review in a particular style.

[1] A strategy that involves identifying the strengths, weaknesses, opportunities and threats within an experience

The examples of questions given in Table 5.3 are only provided as illustrations and you do not need to remember these; the important point is to memorise the 'what, so what, now what' phrase so that it can be used to structure your reflective work.

Table 5.3 Borton's (1970) framework used to guide nursing reflective activity.

What? This is the descriptive level, and all the questions that are asked start with the word what?	**So what?** At this level we look deeper at what is going on behind the experience, to explore it at a theoretical and conceptual level.	**Now what?** Building on the previous level, these questions enable us to consider alternative courses of action and choose the most appropriate.
Example What happened? What did I do? What did others do? What did I feel? What was I trying to achieve? What was good or bad about the experience?	*Example* So what is the importance of this? So what is the significance of this for me? So what more do I need to know about this? So what have I learnt about this?	*Example* Now what could I do? Now what would be the best thing to be? Now what do I need to do? Now what will I do? Now what might be the consequences of this action?

Other techniques are even quicker and easier to use, and can enable you to work with your journal as a 'friend'. For instance, the *three-a-day* technique asks you simply to write a record of your day/experience etc. and identify three aspects of learning that have been achieved. This might simply be 'three things I have learnt today are. . .' or involve more complex ideas such as 'three things I need to find out more about. . .' or 'three things that I need to do as a result of this are. . .'.

Finally, there are the techniques that ask us to analyse our experience against given objectives such as providing evidence of pre-specified *learning outcomes* or *identifying competencies*. These enable us to focus on what we are trying to achieve by working backwards from an end point. It may be that you want to build up a record of your own competency development over the length of your course, in which case separate journal pages for each competency would be a useful and effective structure. Alternatively, you might want to work on developing the evidence base to support learning outcomes for modules you are studying, using your reflective journal as resource material when you are writing an assignment or compiling a portfolio of evidence. The advantages of working towards specific objectives are that you know what it is you are aiming for, and can draw up action plans for achieving this. You can also decide what evidence you will need to demonstrate your objectives in a planned and incremental way, and through using the journal, constantly review how far you are in your schedule of progress.

Creative techniques, on the other hand, are very individualistic and it is unlikely that these would be used where the writing was required as a course component and was going to be read by others, unless the writer chose to share it. *Letter or email writing* in its many forms is a useful strategy for recording emotional experiences, where the writer needs to rid themself of tension before dealing with an incident. *Writing the unsent letter*, for instance, enables the writer to record their feelings as if writing to the person who has instigated them. Often this strategy enables a distance to be created, because the emotional aspects are poured on to the paper, allowing the person to be more rational in dealing with the incident itself. One word of caution with this idea though – when using email to vent your feelings, take care not to push the 'send' button! *Writing with another person in mind* again allows specific viewpoints to be taken, where the writer can defend their position without contradiction, whereas *writing as the other* forces the writer to consider alternative ways of experiencing the event. This can be a useful exercise if you are finding it difficult to get beyond your own emotional responses to something that has happened and need to find a way out of your thought patterns.

Journalistic writing, story telling and poetry writing all enable the writer to be creative in sifting through the contents of the experience and reforming it in a different way that helps them to make sense of it. For instance, imagine yourself as Alistair Cooke writing a 'Letter from America', or as a television reporter sending a broadcast back on the television. Or perhaps consider how Harry Potter would have dealt with that difficult character!

For most of us, the inclination is simply to sit down and start writing a description of an event in a linear form. Others may prefer the order imposed on our thoughts by using a reflective framework that guides us through specific cues in order to explore an incident. Once you have been writing a journal for some time you will find a strategy that suits you best and that you are comfortable with.

However, the suggestions and alternatives above provide examples of the ways that others have used variety in their writing, and devised ways of keeping the journal fresh and dynamic. It may be worth considering experimenting with some of these and seeing what the results are.

This classification is obviously a simplistic one, and is not meant to suggest that the strategies exist in isolation. Indeed, any action will have emotions and feelings associated with it. I have divided them in this way as an illustration of the different foci and outcomes that we might take in our reflective writing, and to emphasise that we can choose from a whole range of ideas depending on what it is we want to achieve and get out of the activity. They provide us with a 'kitbag' of tools that we can select from as appropriate for the jobs that we want them to do.

On-your-own exercise *10 min*

Think about each of the reflective writing strategies in Table 5.2 and answer the following questions about each one in turn:

- What is my initial reaction to this technique – positive, negative, appealing, off-putting, comfortable, uncomfortable etc?
- Why might this be?
- In what ways could I use this technique?
- What sorts of events and experiences within my practice could I use this technique for?
- How could I incorporate strategies for reflective practice within the technique?

Getting started in journal writing

Having thought what you will write about, and how you will approach the writing, the next task is to get started. Unfortunately there is no enlightening advice I can offer about how to start writing. It seems churlish to say 'Just sit down and do it', but that is simply how it is. However, there are various strategies you can adopt to help motivate yourself to write:

(1) It is important to identify your own reasons for wanting to keep a journal, especially if it is not something that you are required to do as part of a course. Look again at the purposes of keeping a journal in Table 5.1 and try to identify those that apply to you. Understanding your motivation, and perhaps writing a reflective piece exploring why you feel the pull to keep a journal, can be the first step to actually starting it (and may be the first piece of writing that goes in the journal!).

(2) Identifying our attitudes to writing and where these have come from may free you up from the rules and boundaries inhibiting your writing.

(3) Establishing a comfortable environment in which to write helps to link writing with relaxation and taking control of the situation. For instance, are you more comfortable writing on a computer than with a pen and paper; or maybe you like to write with a special pen and notebook, or

in a particular place? Perhaps you need to have completed the rest of your daily activities and use specific times in the day to write? Try to think about how you can create an environment to suit yourself that will allow you to start writing.

(4) Identify previous enjoyable experiences of writing and plan to use the elements of these that made them pleasurable. These might be types of writing that you liked (e.g. structured/unstructured, task driven/free flowing etc) and work out how you can plan to use these in your journal. Often, the barriers we put up against starting to write derive from previous experiences that we found stressful, such as examinations or writing essays in our schooldays.

(5) Plan to start simply – perhaps set yourself a target of writing a certain number of words a day, or use the 'three-a-day' technique to review your day and identify significant events and experiences that have happened. Gradually plan to expand what you are doing, and how you are doing it, as you become more comfortable with writing and confident of what you are achieving.

Structuring a journal

At some stage you will need to consider how your journal is going to be organised. At first you may be content to write in a linear fashion, page by page. However, there are other ways in which a diary can be organised, that will facilitate reflective activity and enable you to return to entries and add to your thought processes and learning over time. Some of these are summarised in Table 5.4.

Again, the decisions about the structure of your journal need to arise from your knowledge about yourself – your learning and writing styles, the way you motivate yourself and the ways in which you achieve your objectives in other parts of your life. Try to incorporate these into the structure of your journal, as you are more likely to succeed if you are using familiar tried and tested ways that you are comfortable with.

Ethical issues

Unless required for course work, journals tend to be very private documents. Journaling is under the control of the writer, and a deliberate decision needs to be taken if the entries are to be seen by others. This is not to be undertaken lightly, as many of the entries will be of experiences that have emotional significance for the writer, and/or may be records of incidents where professional misconduct or incidents of questionable quality of care may be recorded.

Nurses are bound by the Code of Professional Conduct (NMC 2002) for the whole of the time they are recorded on the live register of nurses, midwives and health visitors. Thus the decision to show journal entries to others must be taken in the knowledge that professional consequences may ensue if the code of conduct has been contravened. Of course, no one can make you reveal any part of your journal or professional portfolio to others. Where it is

Table 5.4   Some techniques for structuring your journal.

Structure/technique	How it works
The open-page technique	The pages of the book are opened out so the two facing pages are used for each event/experience. The full description is written on the left-hand page in as much detail as possible. The right-hand page is used for reflective activity. The entries are dated, starting with the initial reflection. The pages are returned to at intervals (possibly on a completely random basis), with new reflections being added on an incremental basis, thus developing new insights as the incident itself recedes into the background.
The revolving spiral	This involves exploring an incident using a reflective cycle, such as Gibbs', or Borton's framework for reflection, and creating a reflective review of an incident. The outcome of this will be changed perspective, and probable action that will be taken. Hence, the next time a similar experience occurs it can be explored using the same process, thus creating a continuous spiral of learning through developing expertise and perceptions of a single topic.
Organising a journal through a framework	This is most common when a journal is part of course work and students need to demonstrate learning outcomes such as competencies or a range of experience. Sections can be created for each of these, within which cues are used to facilitate the reflective writing. For instance, a student may use a framework to identify their previous learning and knowledge about a topic, resulting in the identification of specific learning needs, a plan of action to achieve these, identification of the evidence that will be used to support their achievement, and a reflective review of the process.
Focused topic areas	This technique is used where a specific topic is focused on in order to structure the learning to be achieved. Each section in the journal relates to one topic, and is revisited on a regular basis.
Project/research journals and diaries	These are used specifically to keep an on going reflective log of the progress of a project or research study. They enable the researcher to record memos, analytical notes and ideas as the project progresses and develops, thus creating an audit trail.

required to be a public document, you have the choice of what is included in the public part and can remove anything that may result in negative consequences for yourself.

Also, do remember that most of the people with whom you will be sharing your journal will be in a position of authority and are likely to be nurses. They also therefore have a professional responsibility within the code of conduct and may feel the need to take further action about something you have written. They may also facilitate you in considering your own actions and encourage you to seek alternatives or develop what you have done.

Finally, do also remember the need for confidentiality and anonymity regarding any other person who has a part in your journal. This applies to anyone else – patients and their carers, professional workers and your colleagues and educational staff. If you are in any doubt about this, try not to use other people's names at all, or if you do, give them pseudonyms, and make this clear at the beginning of the journal. Another issue to consider, that is related to this, is the use of patient information as evidence or in illustration of your work. Do remember that the Data Protection Act 1998 applies to you, and if you are unclear about your responsibilities within this it is worth checking them out.

On-your-own exercise   *20 min*

Think about the issues raised in this section in relation to creating your own journal.

- What aspects of the Code of Professional Conduct (NMC 2002) do you need to consider when starting your journal?
- Who are you going to be sharing your journal with, and what are the implications of this?
- How would you ensure that you maintained confidentiality and anonymity?
- Do you need to know more about the Data Protection Act 1998 and if so, what are you going to do about it?

Tips for teachers

I believe that, as with most other learning and teaching strategies, the role taken by the educator in facilitating journal writing with students is crucial to its success. I can only pass on some tips that I have learnt over the years, and hope that these may ease your journey and help you to avoid some of the mistakes that I have made before arriving where I am now. These are summarised in Table 5.5.

Conclusion

This chapter has, by necessity, provided a very broad and wide-ranging overview of the use of journals as a learning strategy. It is hoped that students and qualified practitioners alike will be stimulated to try a version of journaling themselves within their professional lives. For many of the nurses I have worked with, the act of journaling brought reflective practice alive and made it, if not an everyday conscious activity, then certainly a regular one. Many have found that journaling enabled them to see the task of constructing a professional portfolio as a dynamic activity, rather than an onerous retrospective, dust-gathering chore. So why not try it out for yourself and see?

Table 5.5   Facilitating others to use journals.

Teacher credibility
Ensure that you are clear about:

- Why you are asking the student to keep a journal
- Your own attitudes towards journaling
- The purpose you want it to serve
- The outcomes you expect it to achieve
- How it will be used as part of your learning and teaching strategy
- The ethical issues involved

A question to think about:

- Is it ethical to ask students to keep a journal if you don't do so yourself?

The nuts and bolts
Think about:

- What type of structure you want the students to use, or whether to leave this to the student
- What the journal will be used for, e.g. assessment, individual tutorials, group work
- How you ensure it will be at the appropriate academic level for the module/course
- Whether it is compulsory
- The style of journal you are using
- Whether it is formative or summative
- How you are going to assess it
- What you are going to assess
- How you can make the marking as straightforward as possible
- Whether you will ask the student to self-assess
- Whether others are to be involved, e.g. mentors

Student preparation
It is worth taking time to:

- Prepare detailed student notes
- Spend a couple of hours briefing the students
- Prepare exemplars and illustrations
- Prepare exercises based on different types of experiences/events
- Prepare exercises using different writing strategies
- Discuss the ethical issues
- Identify what it is you are expecting from students and how it relates to their other work/course outcomes.

Teaching and learning strategies
- It is worth using a learning contract that is negotiated between yourself and the student in terms of outcomes, objectives, structure, action planning and strategies to be used
- Allocate time for individual tutorials so that you can be sure the student understands what is expected of them
- Plan group tutorials/seminars for students to share their experiences of using the journal
- Plan regular review time to ensure that students are using the journal incrementally
- Create milestones so that students have something to aim for, e.g. three-a-day exercises, monthly 500 word summaries, etc.
- Create strategies for self-assessment

NB: Time spent at the beginning in facilitating and supporting students pays dividends at the end

References

Borton, T. (1970) *Reach, Touch, and Teach*. McGraw-Hill, London.

Callister, L.C. (1993) The use of student journals in nursing education: making meaning out of clinical experience. *Journal of Nursing Education*, **32** (4), 185–6.

Cook, I. (2000) Nothing can ever be the case of 'Us' and 'Them' again: exploring the politics of difference through border pedagogy and student journal writing. *Journal of Geography in Higher Education*, **24** (1), 13–27.

Degazon, C.E. & Lunney, M. (1995) Clinical journal: a tool to foster critical thinking for advanced levels of competence. *Clinical Nurse Specialist*, **9** (5), 270–74.

Drevdahl, D.J. & Dorcy, K.S. (2002) Using journals for community health students engaged in group work. *Nurse Educator*, **27** (6), 255–9.

Gibbs, G. (1988) *Learning by Doing. A Guide to Teaching and Learning Methods*. Oxford Polytechnic, Oxford.

Hahnemann, B.K. (1986) Journal writing: a key to promoting critical thinking in nursing students. *Journal of Nursing Education*, **25** (5), 213–15.

Haigh, M.J. (2001) Constructing Gaia: using journals to foster reflective learning. *Journal of Geography in Higher Education*, **25** (2), 167–89.

Holly, M.L. (1988) Reflective writing and the spirit of enquiry. *Cambridge Journal of Education*, **19** (1), 71–80.

Hurtig, W., Yonge, O., Bodnar, D. & Berg, M. (1989) The interactive journal: a clinical teaching tool. *Nurse Educator*, **14** (6), 17, 31, 35.

Jasper, M. (1999) *Assessing and improving student outcomes through reflective writing*. In: *Improving Student Learning Outcomes* (ed. C. Rust). Oxford Centre for Staff Development, Oxford.

Jasper, M. (2003) *Beginning reflective practice*. Nelson Thornes, Cheltenham.

Johns, C. (2000) *Becoming a Reflective Practitioner. A reflective and holistic approach to clinical nursing, practice development and clinical supervision*. Blackwell Science, Oxford.

Landeen, J., Byrne, C. & Brown, B. (1992) Journal keeping as an educational strategy in teaching psychiatric nursing. *Journal of Advanced Nursing*, **17**, 347–55.

Marland, G. & McSherry W. (1997) The reflective diary: an aid to practice-based learning. *Nursing Standard*, **12**, 13–15, 49–52.

Moon, J. (1999a) *Learning Journals*. Kogan Page, London.

Moon, J. (1999b) *Reflection in Learning and Professional Development*. Kogan Page, London.

NMC (2002) *Code of Professional Conduct*. Nursing and Midwifery Council, London.

Perkins, J. (1996) Reflective journals: suggestions for educators. *Journal of Physical Therapy Education*, **10** (1), 8–13.

Rolfe, G., Freshwater, D. & Jasper, M. (2001) *Critical reflection for nursing and the helping professions: a user's guide*. Palgrave, Basingstoke.

UKCC (2001) *The PREP Handbook*. United Kingdom Central Council for Nursing, Midwifery and Health Visiting, London.

Chapter 6

Are You Sitting Uncomfortably? From Group Resistance to Group Reflection in Several Uneasy Moves

Hazel Platzer

Introduction

In this chapter I will explore the reasons why groups may be a powerful and effective way of helping nurses to reflect on their practice in order to develop critical thinking abilities and an experiential knowledge base. I will look at the particular context of nursing which can initially make it difficult for groups to be set up and to work effectively. Such barriers include the ways in which nurses are socialised and educated, and the particular kind of hierarchical systems in which many nurses work, which make it difficult for peers to openly explore their practice and engage in learning from experience. I will also explore the ways in which groups tend to work and how they develop. It is normal for groups to go through stages of development; along the way power struggles and game playing can get in the way of groups working in a productive or useful way. If a group gets 'stuck' at such a stage of development it can become a dangerous or destructive place to be. Other groups move quickly through such stages to become 'working' groups, that is groups where members are really meeting their aims and the members feel they are really getting something valuable from their participation. Finally, I will look at ways in which groups can be set up to increase the likelihood of such success, and I will explore the kinds of skills which facilitators and group members need to develop to make their group work.

The development of these skills will be transferable to other settings outside your group, making you more effective in your teaching, managing and caring roles. They are skills well worth developing whatever your current role, but they do not come easily – the approaches described in this chapter require a commitment to being open enough to learn from experience and this requires learning to tolerate uncertainty and feeling uncomfortable at times. However, you will feel the rewards of doing this through an increased ability to find and offer support in your working environment, and through the satisfaction that comes with continuing to develop your practice.

Why group work could be a good idea in nursing

Using groups to develop work-related skills and knowledge is not a new idea; it is something which goes on informally as part of day-to-day practice in many work settings including nursing. There is a cultural shift towards work-based learning and the concept of learning organisations (Eraut 1994, 1997; Eraut *et al.* 1998; Birchenall 1999; Spouse 2001). Within this there is a move to capitalise on the informal learning that goes on in groups and teams which are part of the work-place, and to make such learning more explicit and valued. This does not mean there is a move to formalise such learning in the sense that it leads to further qualifications or accreditation. Indeed, the converse is true and it is more a case that there is an increasing recognition that much of the expertise and knowledge of professionals can best be developed with the kind of support that can come from group reflection and supervision. Increasingly there is more interest in the use of groups in nursing, with the move towards more formal supervision and recognition of the need for professional development and support (Johns & Graham 1994; Carkhuff 1995; Thomas 1995; Parish *et al.* 1997; Ashford *et al.* 1998; Lee 1999; Arvidsson *et al.* 2001; Martin 2002).

Although not completely synonymous, there is considerable overlap between the intentions, processes and outcomes of supervision and reflective practice (UKCC 1996; Johns 1997; Fowler & Chevannes 1998; Driscoll 2000; Maggs & Biley 2000). Rolfe *et al.* (2001) have suggested that the increased interest in groups is because of resources issues but they also argue that it is mistaken to believe that groups are less resource intensive as facilitators and supervision of facilitators is still required. In the same way that there are different models of reflection and supervision, there are different approaches to running groups for the purposes of facilitating learning from experience. A particular kind of learning in groups, known as action learning sets, has been popular in teacher training and management development for some time (McGill & Beaty 1995) and is also beginning to be adopted within nursing (Graham 1995; Lee 1999; Kirrane 2001).

There are several reasons why group work might be a more effective way of both facilitating reflective practice and providing supervision. Both reflective practice and supervision seek to develop knowledge based on experience and claims are made that both can be educational, restorative (in that they provide support and help to manage stress), and normative (in that they help to maintain good standards) (Butterworth *et al.* 1996; UKCC 1996; Platzer *et al.* 1997; Butterworth *et al.* 1998; Driscoll, 2000). There is accumulating research evidence that individual supervision and methods for promoting reflection do enable such development and support (Johns 1994; White 1996; White *et al.* 1998). However, a number of concerns have been expressed about the individual approach, particularly when only self-directed methods are used, such as journal writing (Richardson 1995; Platzer *et al.* 1997; Scanlan & Chernomas 1997; Cotton 2001). In addition, there are concerns about 'laundering' of reflective journals to fulfill criteria for educational assessment (Wallace 1995), and of course there is always the danger of toxic mentors or incompetent supervisors. An incompetent supervisor is merely someone who lacks the skills that they should bring to their job and they are at worst ineffectual. However, a toxic mentor is one who behaves in a way which undermines the confidence, self-esteem and abilities of the person they are supposed to be helping to develop. These problems in and of themselves are not really a case against individual approaches, as the first can be remedied by taking reflection out of the academic realm (this point will be explored further later in this chapter), and processes for training and managing supervisors should be in place in any organisation.

However, there are more compelling arguments about the potential benefits of reflecting or having supervision in groups. Obvious potential benefits are the effects of peer support, pressure and feedback as well as the shared experience in the group, which is multiplied simply because more people are there (Rolfe *et al.* 2001). A further consideration is the idea that learning is a social process rather than an individual process and this is one of the fundamental beliefs that underpins action learning: that we learn with and from each other in dialogue (McGill & Beaty 1995; Kirrane 2001). Another point which will be explored further in this chapter is that groups remove 'false certainty' (Lyth 1989) and it is only through giving up complete reliance on technical–rational knowledge that we can begin to develop and articulate expert knowledge. Technical–rational knowledge is the kind of scientific knowledge which informs our practice and can easily be verified, i.e. there is clearly a right or wrong way of practising or a 'black and white' answer. This is also sometimes referred to as propositional knowledge. However, there are many areas of practice which are in more of a grey area and where the best approach to take is debatable, less certain and more context dependent. Approaches to developing and articulating expert knowledge rest on a belief that we can find our own answers by problem solving, but also that others can help us arrive at these answers (McGill & Beaty 1995; Driscoll 2000; Johns 2000).

What might get in the way of effective group work?

Whatever arguments are made about the potential benefits of groups, they are by no means straightforward to set up and run effectively. I referred early in this chapter to a general cultural shift towards a learning society and learning organisations. However, if we look specifically at nursing there are many cultural barriers still in place which make the kind of learning offered through reflection difficult to engage in. First and foremost perhaps, it should be said that groups can be dangerous places, particularly if the facilitator is not sufficiently skilled to manage the group dynamics (Rolfe *et al.* 2001). However, even in the hands of a skilled facilitator there are particular cultural barriers to nurses participating in this kind of learning because of the ways in which they have been socialised professionally through their educational and practice experiences (Mountford & Rogers 1996; Johns 1999; Platzer *et al.* 2000b). The hierarchical structure in nursing makes for power inequalities and struggles that make group work difficult (Murrell 1998). Within this, nurses seem to suffer from a form of institutionalised anxiety that is hard to contain in such groups and which increases resistance to working in groups in ways which encourage personal and professional development (Lyth 1989; Maggs & Biley 2000).

The structure provided by the action learning approach seems to be a good way of surmounting this initial anxiety so that groups can develop to the point where they are achieving their aims (Haddock 1997). This approach is explored further in the next section. Another hazard along the way is the propensity for group dynamics to lead to the scapegoating of one particular hapless individual. Whether or not this propensity is more likely in nursing is difficult to know, but it does seem to be a more likely product of a blame culture in nursing in which it is hard to admit to mistakes or ignorance (Oehler & Perault 1986; Lartin 1988). While the very reason for existence of a reflective practice group or supervision group would involve moving away from such a blame culture, it is easy to see how in the early stages of such a cultural shift people in groups need to be in safe hands. Rolfe *et al.* (2001) have made this point quite firmly in their admonitions against groups without facilitators.

Another point worth making, to illustrate both the purpose of reflective or supervision groups and the reasons why there may be difficulties in making them work, is that they deliberately create uncertainty in order to promote learning. It is this probably more than anything, coupled with the ways in which nurses are socialised, that accounts for many of the difficulties experienced in either running a group or being in it. Coping with uncertainty and ambiguity is the key to professional development and learning from experience. Uncertainty pervades professional work (Eraut 1994) and we are often dealing with unique cases for which there are no textbook answers (Schön 1983). However, in a culture where technical–rational or propositional knowledge is prized alongside formal education training and assessment, and where tacit knowledge and experiential knowledge is devalued (Eraut 1997), it is hard for nurses to make the necessary cultural shift to engage in approaches which allow learning from experience. This is doubly difficult where nursing knowledge is further devalued because of the feminisation of the occupation; Johns (1999) has made the point that nurses are particularly disempowered and oppressed because of this. Interesting in this respect is Eraut's (1994) observation that engineers have a public image of a reliable quasi-scientific knowledge base, but in practice they deal with uncertainties by leaving large margins of error and making expert judgements. It would seem that a masculinised occupation does not have the same difficulties in justifying its use of tacit knowledge and lack of propositional knowledge, in spite of the dominant culture which favours propositional knowledge. The point to be made here is that in occupations with high status, which tend to be masculinised or male-dominated, expert knowledge and learning through experience are acceptable, whereas in a feminised occupation such as nursing this same approach can be criticised and taken less seriously on the grounds that it is unscientific.

A final point to make about why groups may be problematic is that there is increasing evidence within nursing that the people running groups do not always have the required skills and experience to facilitate them effectively (Miller *et al.* 1994; Murrell 1998; Dewar & Walker 1999; Johnston & Tinning 2001). This could be particularly problematic when coupled with the kind of hierarchical relationships in nursing which make for power inequalities. In such a system it would be particularly difficult for nurses to confront the issue of lack of facilitation skills in someone perceived to be senior to them in status. However, given that lack of appropriate skill has also been noted in supervisors offering one-to-one supervision (Johns 1999; Heath & Freshwater 2000; Johns, 2001), then perhaps a group at least potentially offers safety in numbers and a better chance of veto! A further problem is that effective questioning skills are required to help people to develop critical thinking skills but there is also evidence that nurse teachers lack sophistication in questioning skills (Sellappah 1998; Phillips & Duke 2001). The barriers to effective group work are summarised in Table 6.1 and some points for potential facilitators to consider are given in Table 6.2. These should be borne in mind when setting up a group or joining a group and can be read in conjunction with the rest of this chapter which sets out ways to overcome these barriers.

Table 6.1   Barriers to effective group work in nursing.

- A hierarchical culture where subordinates are not allowed to question those above them.
- A nurse education system which has not always promoted critical thinking.
- A blame culture where it is hard to be open about and learn from mistakes and where individuals are made into scapegoats.
- Lack of facilitation and effective skills in those in teaching and supervising positions.
- Resistance due to collective anxiety.
- Undue emphasis on formal 'textbook' knowledge and lack of value attached to experiential knowledge.

Table 6.2   Points for facilitators to consider.

- Have you done this before? If not, get an experienced co-facilitator.
- Get yourself a supervisor so you can reflect on your practice as a facilitator.
- Consider using a clear structure such as action learning.
- Develop your questioning skills so that your questions promote critical thinking.
- Remember that you are a facilitator not a leader; if you are doing a lot of the talking in the group you are probably doing something wrong.
- Be prepared to feel uncomfortable some of the time.
- Help the group to maintain a balance of support and challenge.
- Allow silences to happen – they are good opportunities for reflection.

How to set about doing group work

Given the previous discussion about the likely barriers to effective group work in nursing, it is vital that groups are set up and facilitated in such a way that initial resistance can be overcome and participants can see for themselves the potential benefits of such work. We should also take account of the fact that nurses tend to work in hierarchical structures which can make group work difficult. It makes sense therefore to ensure that people in management or mentoring relationships to each other are not members of the same group. It is not absolutely necessary for membership to be fixed (this is known as a closed group) and open groups have been found to work well in providing support in certain settings (e.g. Parish *et al.* 1997). However, it is probably easier in a closed group to develop the kind of trust that is needed for a group to move beyond providing support and also provide an element of challenge which is necessary for reflective learning to take place. The size of a group will also affect this process and ideally reflective practice groups should have about eight members. You should also try to protect the time and space you have, by meeting at a time and in a place where members cannot be interrupted or called out to deal with a crisis. It is also best to try and meet no less than once a fortnight, but preferably once a week.

Setting up useful ground rules

It is standard practice now for people in groups to set out basic ground rules or shared agreements about how they will work together. Such rules usually include maintaining confidentiality, speaking for yourself rather than putting words into other people's mouths or trying to represent them, and treating each other respectfully and non-judgementally. However straightforward these may seem, it is inevitable at some point that such rules will need to be discussed – for instance there will be circumstances when matters disclosed in a group could have implications for the professional accountability of peers in the group. Perhaps the most important thing to establish is that confidentiality will be maintained except in unusual circumstances and then there will still be a commitment from group members to disclose their concerns and intentions. The most important thing about ground rules is that they should be made explicit, and it should be agreed that they can be renegotiated as and when necessary (Rolfe *et al.* 2001). Similarly, both group and individual aims should be made explicit and be negotiated (Rolfe *et al.* 2001). The facilitator needs to be actively engaged in encouraging all members of the group to think about and take responsibility for developing ground rules, rather than simply suggesting a prescribed list or leaving it to chance.

Working effectively with each other

Ground rules such as treating each other respectfully and being non-judgemental sound unambiguous in theory, but in practice it is sometimes hard to know what they mean and it is possible to be unable to know how to act because of them; for instance, it can sometimes be difficult to work out how to give each other feedback and to challenge each other in order to question practice without appearing to give advice or opinions. It is here that the framework for action learning is especially helpful as it provides a clear set of methods for doing just this (McGill & Beaty 1995; Martin 2002). Underlying this set of approaches is a firm belief that learners or practitioners have within them the answers to problems that they need to solve, and that we can help each other to arrive at these through appropriate questioning and feedback, or support and challenge (McGill & Beaty 1995). What we have to do then is avoid well-rehearsed reflection where we appear to be reflecting (Heath & Freshwater 2000). This would be where we were making all the right noises and apparently reflecting, but in a way which was superficial and not challenging ourselves or each other. In order to get beyond this point we have to bring conflict and contradiction to the surface (Johns 1999) and make the familiar unfamiliar (Schön 1983) so that we can move beyond our habitual responses (McGill & Beaty 1995). This brings us back to the point that professional development and reflective learning mean tolerating uncertainty and ambiguity; in our search for answers we have to be prepared to not know the answers and perhaps not arrive at a definite answer or rule that we can apply next time. As already mentioned, there is a clear set of approaches within action learning which will facilitate this; it is the role of both the facilitator and the group members to take responsibility for adhering to these approaches, and from my experience these approaches will show obvious benefits quite quickly. In action learning the idea is that a group should quite quickly become self-facilitating, and an initial function of the facilitator would be to model the kind of behaviour expected in such a group. This would be with a view to making themselves redundant as the members become self-facilitating. Table 6.3 summarises the kind of approaches to interacting with group members to help each other work well in a group together. It is sometimes hard for groups to effectively challenge each other so that they can really reflect. Much of the challenge that is needed to encourage reflection can be done through the use of effective questioning skills. These are summarised in Table 6.4 and considerably more detail can be found in McGill and Beaty (1995) for anyone who feels they need further guidance. As they say, good questions are not ones that make you look clever; they should be:

> 'selfless – [they are not] asked to generate an interesting response or information for the questioner, rather [they are] asked as a way of opening up the presenter's view on their situation.'

> (McGill & Beaty 1995, p.69–70)

Furthermore, however good you become at this, 'sometimes the most supportive and most challenging thing is to say nothing' (McGill & Beaty 1995, p.36). Although there are many useful books to help group members and facilitators develop these skills, the only way to learn how to be in a group or how to facilitate a group is by being in one and reflecting on that experience (Rolfe *et al.* 2001). Hence the importance of having a facilitator who has the appropriate skills to make sure that the group is a safe place, and to act as a positive role model.

The use of effective questioning skills to help people arrive at, or reason out, their own answers is not new and is sometimes referred to as the Socratic method, where question and answer debate was used to tease out philosophical problems.

Table 6.3 How to interact with each other to get the best out of your group.

- Establish clear ground rules which are open to renegotiation.
- Try to help create a supportive and non-competitive atmosphere.
- Remember that reflection is encouraged where there is a good balance between supporting each other and challenging each other.
- Don't give advice – it is usually unhelpful and doesn't help people to problem solve or reflect.
- Listen carefully.
- Attend to how people feel about the event they are describing to you.
- Attend to how people are feeling in the here and now.
- Allow silences so that people have time to think and reflect.
- Don't ask why (this usually feels like an interrogation).
- Avoid the use of closed questions.
- Develop your questioning skills.
- Be prepared to feel uncomfortable sometimes.

Table 6.4 How to challenge members of your group.

- Develop a trusting and supportive atmosphere.
- Remember that all the members of your group have problem-solving abilities; asking the right questions can help each of you do that for yourselves.
- Develop your questioning skills so that your questions make group members explore and think about their practice at a deeper level.
- Question the assumptions that are implicit within people's accounts.
- Ask questions which help members explore how they are feeling now or how they were feeling at the time of the event they are describing.
- Ask open and searching questions which probe or ask for clarification; both will help people to explore their practice at a deeper level.
- Don't give advice but ask questions in such a way that you help people to arrive at their own solutions.
- Remember that challenge is not the same as confrontation or aggression; it's about helping other people to think and reflect, not making them feel attacked or defensive.
- Allow silences to happen – they are good opportunities for reflection.

This dialectic approach goes back to the days of the ancient Greek philosophers and has been recognised as a useful approach in supervision (Overholser 1991). What is perhaps difficult for nurses here is the cultural barrier referred to earlier where people who work in a hierarchical system can find it hard to support and challenge each other as peers. Also they may not previously have had the encouragement to apply intellectual effort to questioning themselves or others (Eraut 1994). Another point to consider here is the effect of hierarchical status on whether or not people feel that they have a right to question each other. McGill and Beaty (1995) have pointed out that those who ask a lot of questions often have higher status or more power than those who have questions posed to them. For nurses then, if they are used to working in a hierarchical system, it may be hard initially in a group to feel entitled to question each other.

How do you know if it is working?

The highest claims made for supervision, reflective practice and adult education are that they are emancipatory, i.e. they can liberate oppressed people, allowing them greater autonomy and empowerment (Freire 1970; Mezirow 1981; Johns 1999; Heath & Freshwater 2000; Platzer *et al.* 2000a; Arvidsson *et al.* 2001; Johns 2001; Glaze 2002). The process of arriving at such emancipation is inevitably uncomfortable as it creates anxiety and disturbs people's world views and taken-for-granted ways of seeing things. So if a group feels very safe and enjoyable we can probably be fairly sure that there is not enough challenge going on in the group to make it work if the aims are to learn through reflection. McGill and Beaty (1995) have made the point that a group can collude to prevent this challenging kind of work and then it becomes too safe and gets stuck; a group that is working enables its members to live with uncertainty or ambiguity.

At this point it is useful to consider the stages that groups go through in their development before they can get to the point of 'working'. Rolfe *et al.* (2001) provide a useful summary of the different models available for understanding the stages that groups go through before they get to the point where they are working in such a way that their aims can be achieved. The first stage is characterised by anxiety and dependency on the facilitator and there is often an expectation that the facilitator will take a leadership role. However, if facilitators do this they will not be enabling the kind of learning that is supposed to be taking place and will quickly find themselves taking the role of expert and advisor; they might just as well be lecturing in that case to a large audience rather than wasting the resources in a small group. When facilitators refuse to take on an expected leadership role they may well find themselves subject to a large dose of hostility and there is usually a power struggle within the group. However, as McGill and Beaty (1995) have noted, it is a role which takes a certain amount of courage. They also point out that attempts at explaining what is going on beyond an initial outline can be counter-productive as people can only learn how to learn in this way by doing it; continual attempts by the facilitator to explain the process can unwittingly put them in a leadership role or intellectualise the process and in so doing stop it from hap-pening. Sooner or later a group should go through further stages where they become more cohesive, trust develops and the group can then get on with the task they have set themselves.

Another useful set of ideas about how groups work can help members and facilitators understand and live with the process they find themselves immersed in. These ideas are about the roles that people take on in groups and the kind of collective defence mechanisms which can operate in groups. Some of these roles and defence mechanisms can lead to a group becoming 'stuck' at an early stage of development and unable to develop into its 'working' phase. Again Rolfe *et al.* (2001) give an accessible account of these and describe how these roles can become problematic. Such roles include those of the 'group jester' who is always making a joke so that nothing serious can be attended to, the 'group harmoniser' who ensures that there is no conflict so nothing difficult ever gets explored, and the 'group patient' who always brings along some interesting work so that others can sit back and avoid looking at their own experience. It is vital to understand that these are roles and not manifestations of people's fixed personalities. Others in the group bear as much responsibility for allowing people to take on these roles as the individual who has taken them on. Everyone in the group is responsible for whether or not the group works and it is easy to collude or become passive and assume that it is just personality and therefore nothing can be done about it. An example of a group defence mechanism is 'pairing' (Bion 1961), where two members of the group form an alliance and a power base, with the rest of the group expecting in some way to be saved by them. In this way the rest of the members do not take responsibility for what is happening in the group but (unconsciously) expect the pair to do all the work and take responsibility. It is important to bear in mind that group roles are not always problematic and can help to keep a group safe and working. Whether roles are destructive or beneficial to the life of the group they are, like defence mechanisms, unconscious, so that people are gen-erally not aware that they have adopted them. This again brings us back to the need for expert facilitation, otherwise groups can be dangerous places (Rolfe *et al.* 2001).

Some thoughts about outcomes and evaluation

If reflection or supervision in groups is emancipatory, then we should expect outcomes indicative of what Mezirow (1981) called perspective transformation and a higher level of critical thinking. Mezirow (1981, p.7) has argued that this is similar to the process of 'conscientisation' described by Freire in which people transcend false consciousness through a problem-posing approach to 'taken-for-granted social roles and expectations and ... habitual ways'. We should also expect to see evidence of an increase in what Eraut (1994) calls professionalism, which includes being part of a self-regulating body with a specialised body of knowledge, primacy of service to the interests of the client, a well-understood value base and the legitimacy of autonomous judgement and independent action. In an evaluation of reflective practice groups on a post-registration diploma in nursing course, some evidence of this kind of transformation was found (Platzer *et al.* 2000a). In this study we found that some nurses identified that they had become:

- less rule-bound
- more able to understand and tolerate the perspectives of others including those both below and above them in the nursing and medical hierarchies
- more confident about their experiential knowledge base
- more able to act confidently in the interests of others
- more able to understand their role within the existing power structures of their organisations.

Their openness to other perspectives, their decreasing certainty in the idea that there are right or wrong answers, and their increased ability to tolerate uncertainty, suggest that as a result of their learning through reflective practice groups, they had developed the ability to think critically (Brookfield 1987) and had reached the higher stages of the reflective learning cycle (Boud *et al.* 1985). Such perspective transformation allows people to deal with others in a fair and equitable manner (FitzGerald 1994). Another recent study reported similar outcomes from group supervision with reported increases in autonomy, professional identity, confidence, assertiveness, self-esteem, reduced stress and burn-out and an integration of theoretical and practical knowledge with a more holistic and empathic understanding of patients (Arvidsson *et al.* 2001).

Although action learning sets, group supervision and reflective practice groups seem to be increasingly common in nursing, there have been very few published evaluations. However, we should be wary of applying a set of parameters which are inappropriate for measuring what is going on. In much the same way that reflection and supervision are supposed to help us access those parts of our knowledge base which are tacit and experiential, so methods of evaluation should be appropriate for the measurement of such processes. Reflective practice has developed because of the limits of technical–rational knowledge for professional practice; any research into it must therefore logically steer away from empiricist approaches. Qualitative research within a critical realist paradigm is the most appropriate way to evaluate what is going on. In addition, we have a wealth of experiential knowledge of how groups work from many years of their use in therapy, counselling and the personal growth movement.

This caution about research methods is offered because there is a real danger that the whole value and purpose of the reflective practice movement in nursing will be lost as it is hijacked by assessors and rational-technocrats. Johns (1999, 2001) and Heath and Freshwater (2000) have made the point that within supervision, because of the culture within nursing, there is a real danger that supervisors will have a technical interest in supervision which serves to manage the anxiety of the institution rather than being empowering or emancipatory for the practitioner. Such approaches will not work in a way that brings tacit knowledge to the fore and can serve as instruments of surveillance and counter-reflection (Johns 1999; Gilbert 2001).

A final point to make here is, I believe, that reflection and supervision have to be removed from any association with the assessment of formal learning. Once nurses are assessed and accredited for their ability to reflect we immediately constrain their ability and potential to take the kinds of risks which are associated with reflective learning. How can registered nurses begin to tolerate uncertainty and live with the idea that there are no right or wrong answers if reflection is 'taught' in an environment where they have to produce written evidence of their ability to reflect? How many of the increasing number of reflective practice modules on post-registration courses actually develop students' ability to reflect through experiential learning, and how many formally teach about reflection and assess the students' learning at the end by a written essay? McGill and Beatty have made this point very strongly:

> 'The logic of developing the learner as a learner, the reflective practitioner and the competent graduate conflicts in logic, and in spirit, with an assessment system which is controlled, implemented and validated separately from the learner.'
>
> (McGill & Beaty 1995, p.246)

If we are witnessing a trend where reflective practice is assessed in this way, then it is probably symptomatic of the continuing lack of confidence within the profession to assert the legitimacy of our experiential knowledge base. It is also symptomatic of a general trend that much of the formal learning which takes place in higher education settings does not really prepare practitioners, and the situation has been made worse by the current inexorable adoption of modularisation which further fragments knowledge (Eraut 1997). This is not to say that reflection should not be built into formal learning opportunities, but as Birchenall (1999) has said, we need to enhance work-based learning opportunities and rethink the relationship between institutions of higher education and service provision.

Conclusion

I hope this chapter has set out reasons why it might be worth the effort of setting up and participating in a group for reflection and/or supervision. Although some elements of the chapter imply it might be a complicated process, other parts show that it is really only an extension of what many of us already do. However, setting it up can help those processes to become more efficient and make sure that everyone gets a chance to benefit from the support and challenge which group work can offer. Eraut *et al.* (1998) have made the point that a lot of informal learning takes place in work settings but that such learning often takes a lot longer than it needs to. McGill and Beaty (1995) say that action learning accelerates the kind of support that people normally offer each other. Given that Spouse (2001) has observed that it takes ten years to become an expert, it seems sensible to use any method we can to help progress development. Johns (1994, p.119) has observed that many practitioners would prefer to stick to routine and ritual practice rather 'than face the effort of curiosity, reflection and commitment'. For anyone who doubts whether or not groups are worth the effort, then the final words should go to a nurse who participated in a reflective practice group on a post-registration course and had this to say afterwards:

> 'Then I thought well, if I can gain from people teaching me what the better route would be then (I) have to go through a bit of anguish myself, and give something to the group so that (I) can actually get something back for myself – but certainly the very first few groups it was very difficult ... I think the people that were in the group I was in were quite enthusiastic to try ... the six months to start with were probably hell and the next six months we actually gained something from it and we knew what it was and I think at the end of it we'd have liked the group itself to have continued outside of college.
>
> (Platzer *et al.* 2000b, p.1007)

Acknowledgements

Thanks to all the students on the Diploma in Professional Studies in Nursing (DPSN) at University College Chichester (formerly Chichester Institute of Higher Education) who participated in the evaluation of reflective practice groups which inspired this chapter. Thanks also to Caroline Davies and Roo Wheeler, practice development nurses in Brighton and Sussex Universities Hospital Trust, for insightful discussions on the current state of reflective and supervision groups in practice.

References

Arvidsson, V., Lofgren, H. & Fridlund, B. (2001) Psychiatric nurses' conceptions of how a group supervision programme in nursing care influences their professional competence: a 4-year follow-up study. *Journal of Nursing Management*, 9, 161–71.

Ashford, D., Blake, D., Knott, C., Platzer, H.K. & Snelling, J. (1998) Changing conceptions of reflective practice in social work, health and education: an institutional case study. *Journal of Interprofessional Care*, 12, 7–19.

Bion, W.R. (1961) *Experiences in Groups and Other Papers*. Tavistock, London.

Birchenall, P. (1999) Developing a work-based learning philosophy. *Nurse Education Today*, 19, 173–4.

Boud, D., Keogh, R. & Walker, D. (1985) *Reflection: Turning Experience into Learning*. Kogan Page, London.

Brookfield, S.D. (1987) *Developing Critical Thinkers.* Open University, Milton Keynes.

Butterworth, T., Bishop, V. & Carson, J. (1996) First steps towards evaluating clinical supervision in nursing and health visiting. 1. Theory, policy and practice development. A review. *Journal of Clinical Nursing,* 5, 127–32.

Butterworth, T., Faugier, J. & Burnard, P. (1998) *Clinical Supervision and Mentorship in Nursing,* Stanley Thornes, Cheltenham.

Carkhuff, M. (1995) Reflective learning: work groups as learning groups. *Journal of Continuing Education in Nursing,* 27, 209–14.

Cotton, A.H. (2001) Private thoughts in public spheres: issues in reflection and reflective practices in nursing. *Journal of Advanced Nursing,* 36 (4), 512–19.

Dewar, B. J. & Walker, E. (1999) Experiential learning: issues for supervision. *Journal of Advanced Nursing,* 30, 1459–67.

Driscoll, J. (2000) Clinical supervision: a radical approach, *Mental Health Practice,* 3, 8–10.

Eraut, M. (1994) *Developing Professional Knowledge and Competence.* The Falmer Press, London.

Eraut, M. (1997) Perspectives on defining 'The Learning Society'. *Journal of Education Policy,* 12, 551–8.

Eraut, M., Alderton, J., Cole, G. & Senker, P. (1998) Learning from other people at work. In: *Learning at Work* (ed. F. Coffield). Policy Press, Bristol.

FitzGerald, M. (1994) Theories of reflection in nursing. In: *Reflective Practice in Nursing* (eds A. Palmer, S. Burns & C. Bulman) pp. 63–84. Blackwell Science, Oxford.

Fowler, J. & Chevannes, M. (1998) Evaluating the efficacy of reflective practice within the context of clinical supervision. *Journal of Advanced Nursing,* 27, 379–82.

Freire, P. (1970) *Pedagogy of the Oppressed,* Herter and Herter, New York.

Gilbert, T. (2001) Reflective practice and clinical supervision: meticulous rituals of the confessional. *Journal of Advanced Nursing,* 36, 199–205.

Glaze, J. (2002) Reflection as a transforming process: student advanced nurse practitioners' experiences of developing reflective skills as part of an MSc programme. *Journal of Advanced Nursing,* 34, 639–47.

Graham, I. W. (1995) Reflective practice: using the action learning group mechanism. *Nurse Education Today,* 15, 28–32.

Haddock, J. (1997) Reflection in groups: contextual and theoretical considerations within nurse education and practice. *Nurse Education Today,* 17, 381–5.

Heath, H. & Freshwater, D. (2000) Clinical supervision as an emancipatory process: avoiding inappropriate intent. *Journal of Advanced Nursing,* 32, 1298–306.

Johns, C. (1994) Reflective Practice in Nursing. A guided reflection (eds A. Palmer, S. Burns & C. Bulman), pp. 174–81.

Johns, C. (1997) Reflective practice and clinical supervision, part 2: guiding learning through reflection to structure the supervision 'space'. *European Nurse,* 2, 192–204.

Johns, C. (1999) Reflection as empowerment? *Nursing Inquiry,* 6, 214–49.

Johns, C. (2000) *Becoming a Reflective Practitioner: A Reflective and Holistic Approach to Clinical Nursing, Practice Development and Clinical Supervision.* Blackwell Science, Oxford.

Johns, C. (2001) Depending on the intent and emphasis of the supervisor, clinical supervision can be a different experience. *Journal of Nursing Management,* 9, 139–45.

Johns, C. & Graham, J. (1994) The growth of management connoisseurship through reflective practice. *Journal of Nursing Management,* 2, 253–60.

Johnston, A. & Tinning, R. (2001) Meeting the challenge of problem-based learning: developing the facilitators. *Nurse Education Today,* 21, 161–9.

Kirrane, C. (2001) Using action learning in reflective practice. *Professional Nurse,* 16, 1102–5.

Lartin, J.M. (1988) Scapegoating: identifying and revealing the process. *Journal of Nursing Administration*, **18**, 25–31.

Lee, N. (1999) Thinking reflectively: solutions through action learning. *Nursing Times*, **95**, 54–5.

Lyth, Menzies. I. (1989) *The Dynamics of the Social: selected essays, Volume 2*. Free Association Books, London.

Maggs, C. & Biley, A. (2000) Reflections on the role of the nursing development facilitator in clinical supervision and reflective practice. *International Journal of Nursing Practice*, **6**, 192–5.

Martin, V. (2002) Developing and working in a group. *Nursing Management UK*, **8**, 28–31.

McGill, I. & Beaty, L. (1995) *Action Learning: A guide for professional, management and educational development*. Kogan Page, London.

Mezirow, J. (1981) A critical theory of adult learning and adult education. *Adult Education*, **32**, 3–24.

Miller, C., Tomlinson, A. & Jones, M. (1994) *Learning Styles and Facilitating Reflection*. English National Board for Nursing, Midwifery and Health Visiting, London.

Mountford, B. & Rogers, L. (1996) Using individual and group reflection in and on assessment as a tool for effective learning. *Journal of Advanced Nursing*, **24**, 1127–34.

Murrell, K. (1998) The experience of facilitation in reflective groups: a phenomenological study. *Nurse Education Today*, **18**, 303–9.

Oehler, J.M. & Perault, P.Z. (1986) The process of scapegoating in a neonatal nurses' group. *Group*, **10**, 74–84.

Overholser, J.C. (1991) The Socratic method as a technique in psychotherapy supervision. *Professional Psychology – Research and Practice*, **22**, 68–74.

Parish, C., Bradley, L. & Franks, V. (1997) Managing the stress of caring in ITU: a reflective practice group. *British Journal of Nursing*, **6**, 1192–6.

Phillips, N. & Duke, M. (2001) The questioning skills of clinical teachers and preceptors: a comparative study. *Journal of Advanced Nursing*, **33**, 523–9.

Platzer, H.K., Blake, D. & Ashford, D. (2000a) An evaluation of process and outcomes from learning through reflective practice groups on a post-registration nursing course. *Journal of Advanced Nursing*, **31**, 689–95.

Platzer, H.K., Blake, D. & Ashford, D. (2000b) Barriers to learning from reflection: a study of the use of groupwork with post-registration nurses. *Journal of Advanced Nursing*, **31**, 1001–8.

Platzer, H.K., Snelling, J. & Blake, D. (1997) Promoting reflective practitioners in nursing: a review of theoretical models and research into the use of diaries and journals to facilitate reflection. *Teaching in Higher Education*, **2**, 103–21.

Richardson, R. (1995) Humpty Dumpty: reflection and reflective nursing practice. *Journal of Advanced Nursing*, **21**, 1044–50.

Rolfe, G., Freshwater, D. & Jasper, M. (2001) *Critical Reflection for Nursing and the Helping Professions: A User's Guide*. Palgrave, Basingstoke.

Sampson, E. & Marthas, E. (1991) *Group Process for the Health Professions*. Delmar Publishers, New York.

Scanlan, J.M. & Chernomas, W.M. (1997) Developing the reflective teacher. *Journal of Advanced Nursing*, **25**, 1138–43.

Schön, D.A. (1983) *The Reflective Practitioner*. Basic Books, London.

Sellappah, S. (1998) The use of questioning strategies by clinical teachers. *Journal of Advanced Nursing*, **28**, 142–8.

Spouse, J. (2001) Work-based learning in health care environments. *Nurse Education in Practice*, **1**, 12–18.

Thomas, P. (1995) A study of the effectiveness of staff support groups. *Nursing Times*, **91**, 36–9.

UKCC (1996) *Position Statement on Clinical Supervision for Nursing and Health Visiting,* United Kingdom Central Council for Nursing, Midwifery and Health Visiting, London.

Wallace, D. (1995) The use of reflective diaries for formative assessment: A critical analysis. In: *Macmillan Open Learning Reflective Practice Conference.* Commonwealth Centre, London.

White, E. (1996) Clinical supervision and Project 2000: the identification of some substantive issues. *Nursing Times Research*, **1**, 102–11.

White, E., Butterworth, T. & Bishop, V. (1998) Clinical supervision: insider reports of a private world. *Journal of Advanced Nursing*, **28**, 185–92.

Chapter 7

Teachers' and Students' Perspectives on Reflection-on-Action

Chris Bulman

Introduction

From responses to past editions of this book, it is evident that nurses are keen to know more from students and teachers who are involved in teaching and learning about reflection-on-action. If you are faced with the task of introducing a more reflective education as a teacher, or with the request to try out some reflection as a student, then being able to access other opinions and experiences from 'the horse's mouth' may well be a useful place to start.

In the past we have focused on the student perspective more than any other, concentrating on the need to provide handy support and advice for any nurse embarking on reflection for the first time (Holms & Stephenson 1994; Bulman & Burns 2000). However, readers have brought to our attention that teachers would appreciate the chance to access the practical knowledge of others who have developed some experience in teaching and facilitating reflection with nurses; thus the inclusion of both students' and teachers' perspectives in this chapter.

Group discussion

Teachers from a variety of different health care programmes and undergraduate pre-registration adult field students from Oxford Brookes University's School of Health and Social Care were invited to take part in two separate focus groups in order to give them the opportunity to share their attitudes, perceptions and opinions about reflection. (In the previous edition we focused on post-registration students' experiences; for this edition we felt it was timely to talk to pre-registration undergraduates.) Permission was gained to tape record the focus groups rather than rely on note taking, thus creating a more relaxed and spontaneous environment for group discussion. The tapes produced were transcribed, reflected on and then organised into themes relating to the two discussion areas below. Hopefully you will be able to recognise many of the concerns and issues raised and validate them through your own personal experiences, as well as identifying the points that affect these accounts; such aspects as the particular people who volunteered to talk about their experiences, the influences of 'group speak', and my own influences as the organiser of the focus groups, as well as my reflection and interpretation of their discussions.

Focus group discussion concentrated on the following areas:

(1)   What reflection means to teachers and students
(2)   Their experiences of teaching and learning about reflection.

The aim was to promote a free-flowing discussion where ideas, beliefs and issues could be responded to openly between group members. Prompts were used to encourage people to share more and to get them to talk when issues came up that seemed valuable to explore further. As group members relaxed and discussion got underway, they were enthusiastic about sharing their thoughts and experiences and providing an insight into the realities of teaching and learning about reflection. This work, along with past focus group work (Bulman & Burns 2000), provides some fundamental insights into the concerns and experiences of teachers and students. I have presented the themes that emerged from teachers' and students' discussions illustrated by their narrative, and have also related these themes back to the literature and research so that you can see the links and contradictions between them. While this is not research at the moment, it represents some valuable evaluation material for us as educationalists; I hope you find it useful too.

Focusing on teachers

How teachers see reflection

Teachers viewed reflection as a strategy or tool for learning, as a chance to think back over practice experiences and explore feelings, or the emotional component of learning. Reflection was seen as a useful tool in teaching, in finding out what students had learnt and what they felt about it; as a way to start thinking 'what have I learnt?'.

Teachers recognised the potential of reflection to provide a reciprocal link between theory and practice and there was a sense that teaching students about reflection gave them a 'lifeline' with which they could begin to make sense of their practice.

A teacher talking about preparing students for their first clinical placements:

'It was a case of what can we give these students (in practice), that will enable them to make sense of the little bit of material that we have taught them.'

'The least they could do would be to frame a couple of questions which would perhaps make them feel more safe in the middle of London, in a mental health placement on the Isle of Dogs, having to cope with the homeless, you know miles away from any level of "safety".'

Teachers recognised the importance of the past experiences of students in influencing their reflective ability and in giving them confidence that they knew something about the world:

'To know that what they've done in the past has some relevance to what they do now, you can really pull that out in the reflective process.'

'Their personal experience of anything will influence their subsequent learning.'

There were concerns about traditional ways of education and nurse training that had influenced people's ability to be creative and be independent learners:

'There's something about creative ability and I'm wondering if sometimes, with older people and the original way they were nursing, whether we got rid of that, that we didn't value creativity and we weren't taught to be problem solvers.'

The effects of past educational experiences and working culture are raised in studies by Mountford and Rogers (1996), Francis *et al.* (1998), Platzer *et al.* (2000a) and Glaze (2001b), emphasising the importance of exploring and taking into account people's experiences and how they shape and influence the way that we perceive and adjust to adult centred learning, typified by reflection.

There was also a feeling among teachers that reflective education was not a fast track process, but something that took time, characterised by gradual professional growth. Hallett (1997) links this gradual development with practice, suggesting that reflection stems from the need to focus on the nature and quality of professional knowledge, recognising that professional education is more than acquiring skills and facts but also involves the development of clinical expertise and know-how that develops from practice. Additionally Mallik (1998) and Durgahee (1996) suggest that reflection is not an automatic process but requires encouragement, reinforcement, supervision and training, again suggesting a gradual developmental process.

'I think it works (as a tool for learning) but it takes a long time for it to become a rich learning tool.'

'I think that people will only do it when they're individually ready for it. So I think we can do what we can to share things from our perspective but sometimes that can put people off because they feel they're different or whatever.'

Introducing and incorporating reflection

Teachers used various ways to introduce and incorporate reflection in their teaching; however, there was an agreement that it cannot just be an 'add on'; that reflection needs to be incorporated into a course philosophy and discussed and planned into a programme to become meaningful and useful:

'You can't just teach it as a theoretical thing, there has to be some activity built in, starting from where they're at.'

'It's something that requires each person to click, which is really difficult to assess in academic terms. I think it is a professional versus academic tension as to how you manage that.'

'Maybe students need to know from the beginning that it's a journey, that it's not going to end, that they're going to build on and learn from these experiences; it's not something that they can complete in a module.'

People generally began with sessions giving information about reflection, trying to 'sell' the concept, using theory, but also making use of practical ways to get them to start thinking about reflection and the skills necessary for reflection:

'I usually say look I'm going to put it all before you, have a go, try, but don't worry if it doesn't click straightaway or if you don't know what the heck I'm talking about.'

Reactions to these introductory sessions were not always positive:

'What are we doing this for, it isn't nursing?'

'What on earth's she on about?'

There were concerns about those who came from a very structured work environment, or who had experienced other more structured courses; teachers felt they could find it difficult to be given the freedom to be self-directed. It was clear that teachers recognised that people came from a variety of backgrounds and that time was usefully spent in sorting out group dynamics, and teaching people how to learn from each other and 'pull each other along'.

Facilitating students

A number of research studies suggest the fundamental importance of effective facilitation in the development of reflection (Stoddart *et al.* 1996; Francis *et al.* 1998; Page & Meerabeau 2000; Platzer *et al.* 2000b; Paget 2001). Considering learning generally, Rogers (1983) also stresses the importance of the relationship between facilitator and learner, and Bolton (2001) focuses on the importance of the teacher's role in developing trust, respect, openness, confidence and security in the facilitation of reflection. Such a vision of facilitative teaching appears to be a lot to live up to, but as Bolton points out, the relationship between student and facilitator just needs to be 'good enough', and if we get it wrong we can always learn from our mistakes!

Over time, the focus group teachers were aiming to get students to develop a sense of how they could learn, encouraging them to write in journals, portfolios and reflective essays and to develop skills through experiential learning as well as through action learning groups, class discussions and working with mentors and practice link lecturers. Things did not always go smoothly and students did not always conform to the adult learner mode:

'Sometimes it works and sometimes it goes completely flat doesn't it... we find there are lots of peaks and troughs in the term.'

'Sometimes they can't be bothered with problem solving, they would rather have it on a plate.'

'I'm not confident that they use it [reflective portfolio] as a learning tool, in the way perhaps we hope they would.'

The issues of time, the impact of the practice link lecturer and the skills of the mentor were all mentioned as factors that could impede the use of good reflection:

'There aren't enough people out there who are skilled in reflection to facilitate some of the learning that could come from that [reflective portfolios].'

One teacher talked specifically about the issue of keeping a diary, saying that she didn't keep a diary regularly but only did it for a particular purpose. This got others thinking about the issue of motivating students to see the benefits of reflective writing:

'That could be a loophole in my teaching that somehow, I need to help students decide if a diary is going to be useful.'

Concerns were also expressed about the quality of reflection that students were able to produce in their diaries and the dilemma of keeping diaries confidential, when students would probably benefit from some facilitation of their writing skills. In Chapter 5 Melanie Jasper picks up on many of the concerns expressed here by teachers, and offers some possible solutions. Additionally, although nursing research suggests that students appear to find the use of reflective journals helpful, it is unclear whether they support the development of deeper levels of critical thinking, and there are issues surrounding the assessment of what constitutes private diaries (McCaugherty 1991; Landeen *et al.* 1995; Richardson & Maltby 1995; Shields 1995; Clarke & Graham 1996; Durgahee 1996; Riley-Doucet & Wilson 1997; Wong *et al.* 1997; Fonteyn & Cahill 1998).

There was a suggestion that people may not view themselves as reflective but that it may be that people just reflect differently depending on their learning styles:

'I don't know if people reflect differently; maybe they emphasise a different bit depending on their learning style.'

The issue of learning styles (Honey & Mumford 1986) linked to reflection is not one that has generally been pursued by nurse researchers. Spencer and Newell (1999) did collect information on learning styles from participants in their quasi-experimental pilot study; however, they did not publish these particular findings as part of their research report. The point raised above by teachers would therefore be useful to investigate further.

Teachers also recognised the importance of the environment and the situation on people's ability to be reflective. They related examples of how they worked out where students were with reflection and what they knew:

'I always look at their experiences of reflection so far; many have come across it before.'

'... I get them to move then, on to a different level, to critique it really, to look at the strengths and limitations of using reflection.'

'Some of them in the past seem to have been sold it as the "be all and end all" of learning about experience.'

'The thing is finding out what they understand by it and sharing experiences.'

There was also a sense that people could be easily put off by the word 'reflection':

'You need to talk about it more broadly; just mentioning the word can put people off, like the nursing process!'

The need to link reflection with research was also noted – in the teaching of qualitative approaches, through the promotion of reflexivity, thinking about the self as researcher and even using reflection in a research design.

The teachers' discussions encompassed a broad range of issues involved in the facilitation of reflection, from writing to research, from individual concerns to environmental and organisational influences. Teachers were very aware of the pros and cons involved in facilitating reflection, and their own experiences of using reflection appeared to be influential in understanding things from a student's perspective.

Teachers talking about their own experiences as students:

'I hated it at the time ... now I've learnt what it means and how to use it.'

'We'd sit in silence; the guy had an unstructured facilitation approach and I just thought what a complete waste of time... I thought I'd much rather be over the road shopping...'

Being a reflective teacher

Despite the difficulties that get in the way of reflection, as mentioned above, teachers were very positive about the process. They liked to use their own experiences and humour to get things across to students. It was suggested that students were able to pick up when teachers obviously didn't believe in reflection themselves:

'There's a bit of a perception around that some teachers are not themselves reflective, and that therefore they are teaching an approach that they haven't experienced.'

'If you're going to teach it, it is important to reflect or have some strategy as a reflector.'

Teachers were aware of the importance of self-disclosure, of simply saying what you do yourself and being honest.

'I think that it adds credibility if you are reflective and if you have a belief in it. Students are very quick to see through you if you don't have belief behind it.'

Scanlan and Chernomas (1997), Duke (2000) and Hyrkas *et al.* (2001) highlight the benefits of having experience in reflection if you are involved in teaching and are facilitating reflection; indeed Duke would go as far as to say that to understand reflection it needs to be lived and experienced. Mallik (1998), however, suggests that teachers may not necessarily be committed to developing themselves through reflection. Additionally Scanlan *et al.* (2002) found in their study of teachers that personal reflective abilities did not necessarily transfer to the classroom and that it was experienced teachers who were more confident using reflection in the classroom. They also suggest that class size and teachers' emotions while teaching also influenced classroom reflections; however, there are some design limitations with this study which are discussed in Chapter 1.

The right messages and the dilemma of boundaries

Teachers also had concerns about their own abilities to 'get their message across' and to create a positive experience for the students. These comments seem to relate to many of the issues raised above concerning facilitation:

> 'I sometimes worry that I might be trying to facilitate reflection among students, but actually they feel a bit threatened because they're not quite sure why I'm posing the question that I do.'

> 'I'm quite careful to put boundaries on it and I say to them look, I don't want this to be an exercise in psychodrama or psychotherapy.'

There was a sense that keeping things in perspective and not letting them spiral out of control was important, and a realisation that after reflective sessions people have to get on with their everyday lives. However, there was also a sense that sometimes it is necessary to step outside boundaries and push people on a little more:

> 'Sometimes those big "ahas" come and it turns the whole placement around from a complete nightmare to something they know they can do.'

Teachers also realised the need to support people in choosing what might be worth reflecting on for an assignment, helping them to choose something worthwhile and tangible, to avoid students getting frustrated and wasting their time 'splitting hairs' or pursuing something that was not going to be worthwhile.

Teachers were able to offer a variety of ideas and perspectives on teaching based on their own experiences. There were some useful insights into encouraging students to reflect on difficult as well as everyday experiences, and using reflection as a process to raise issues from practice. There was also a sense that teachers were developing their abilities to get students to think about 'making the ordinary, extraordinary' (Atkins & Murphy 1993; Bolton 2001):

> 'It's much easier to reflect on a difficult incident than on things that are going right, which actually would be so productive and of value, but you have to drag it out of them.'

> 'The natural human instinct is to focus on difficult issues, not on what really goes well, because if it goes really well you do something different like go out for a drink or whatever!'

> 'I often choose half a dozen really ordinary things, taking blood, putting in a Venflon, cleaning someone up, very simple things to get them to think hard about what goes through their mind, when they're doing those sorts of things for

patients. So tasks have really got a lot of mileage in them; what you're going to do to another human being. I get them to stick it up on the wall and share it between them; they get so much buzz out of it.'

'You're really getting them to challenge what they take for granted, something that might be ritualistic practice. Then they can see the value of reflective practice, they can see what I'm getting at. It's a way of illustrating what I'm talking about.'

Others also used 'everyday tasks' to encourage students to think more critically about their practice, for example making a bed:

'You can see the student start to see, I know what this is about now and heads start to nod and it does start to make sense to them. I think the challenge then is whether they actually go out and do it in practice.'

Giving students signposts and an information base about reflection was also seen as important:

'Students feed back that they find it very valuable to get a clear understanding of all the terminology that's involved in reflection and critical incidents. What makes an incident critical, what does analysis mean and all the skills of synthesis?'

'I've facilitated some sessions on reflection in writing, showing examples in terms of description and then theory integration and the way action planning arises from reflection... I don't know if the students were necessarily able to write in a more reflective way afterwards.'

'Sometimes people's natural way of thinking is very structured and they do find checklists like Chris Johns' and cycles very useful.'

'You need to look at the expectations of your group and make sure everyone's on the same wavelength.'

Seeing students develop

Teachers seemed to draw on their experiences with students to inform their own judgements about reflection:

'They said they hated it at first but by the time they finished the course they realised the benefits of it.'

'People really like reflecting in action learning groups.'

'Since starting the programme and being introduced to reflection in the context of nursing, it started to click and she writes really well in a reflective way and is the type of student I think we'd all really want.'

'Old students come back to train as mentors. You can see that they've really got it; they're really keen to facilitate it in others. It's a real gosh! These people have really moved on since we taught them as first years. They value it, do it and encourage students to do it.'

Commitment and challenge

Teachers also had concerns about students' commitment to reflection. While they wanted to promote a different way of thinking about and valuing practice, they wondered whether students were able to do it:

'Something's got to click and make a connection.'

'There's the odd occasion when you think I'm not quite sure whether this has ever clicked.'

'Does that person actually use reflection or are they paying lip service to it?'

The teachers also shared some useful experiences on facilitation and the need to support and encourage people as well as challenge them:

'To start with you need to be patient; they may ramble, chuck loads at you which isn't particularly reflective...'

'The worst thing in the world is when you think you've got to say something really important. They need to be able to make mistakes and say anything.'

'Having fun reflecting with other people can encourage them to have a go.'

'Sometimes I think reflection conjures up a rather solitary lonely activity and it's trying to think of other approaches, not just writing a diary or whatever.'

Teachers' discussions seemed to communicate a sense of their commitment to making practice and theory equally important and to encouraging nurses to think critically about their practice; to get in touch with their feelings about their work and to look at their ability to change and develop for the benefit of their clients. There was a continued sense that developing reflection is not a 'quick fix' process; but that you need to make a purposeful start knowing that it may take some time for students to recognise and appreciate reflection on their experiences.

Focusing on students

How students see reflection

The students had a great deal to say about what reflection meant to them. It was seen as a process of self-development, as challenging and analysing experiences and as a link between theory and practice. They focus on cognition here, but later when prompted discuss the emotional and active elements of reflection:

'For me it's a means of self-development, of spiritual growth I suppose.'

'To me it's basically linking theory to practice; thinking about my practice. I would say it is thinking critically, but not thinking in an abstract way, but thinking about experience; this is how I see it.'

'It's about challenging what you've done, how you affect other people, how you could do things better.'

'I've always questioned things and analysed stuff anyway and then to come here and find out that is what you want us to do, I've not found it hard to adjust.'

Students expressed a sense of commitment to the process of reflection and to improving themselves as nurses and as people:

'It's about self-fulfilment; I've read through my reflections and felt so chuffed about it. How you feel yourself when you come to some realisation from reflection; you don't need other people to mark it in an essay. It's about improving your own practice.'

'It's very difficult to change what you do and how you behave in any other way. I wouldn't know how else you could do it; rather than getting them to look at what you do and analysing it, seeing how you could do it better and raising people's self-awareness in effect.'

'It's about improving self-awareness, learning in a way which is not just reading and memorising. It's about relating it to practice and yourself. It's linked to self-awareness but also to self-learning, where I can direct my learning. I choose what I can reflect on. It's linked to being aware of my "holes in practice"; it is in a way empowering me as a person, as a nurse, giving me responsibility for my learning and developing my ability to know what we should know. I find this course in a way kind of personality building.'

These comments equate with nursing research findings exploring reflection-on-action, for instance Jasper (1999) reports the facilitation of personal development in her ongoing study of reflective writing; participants changed and developed as people and developed their analytical and critical skills which impacted on their practice. Durgahee (1996) and Clarke and Graham (1996) also report developments in students' ability to question and challenge practice, and Shields (1995) reports students improved problem solving, personal development and self-analysis.

Drawing on personal experiences

Students shared their past experiences and how they felt these had affected their current views and experiences of reflection. One student's past experiences clearly reflected traditional styles of education in which he had obviously felt capable but he expressed a sense of frustration and dissatisfaction:

'I was always taught to listen, read and memorise every subject. I have always studied subjects which in a way were good for that kind of teaching – Latin and Greek in High School, Engineering with a lot of Mathematics; not applied except in the dissertation.'

'On the job [engineering] there is hierarchy, not self-directed learning, it is not personality building it is personality destroying.'

His experiences described above differed greatly from his experiences on a nursing course where he had encountered practice almost straight away and he had enjoyed a more liberal, reflective style of education. He appeared to value the opportunity for self-directed learning and the opportunity to flourish as a person as well as a professional.

Another student left school early and did A levels as a mature student; she described A levels as:

'Having some analysis but there was not much learning about what I thought.'

She described her alternative hippie-style traveller's life before she had come back into education, commenting on the effects of this alternative culture and how the course was an extension of this. She hadn't found the transition difficult:

'The travelling way of life is very reflective.'

Both of these students were mature and had life and education experience which had shaped their attitude to learning; this is evidently not the case for all students (Platzer *et al.* 2000a,b). The purpose of a reflective education is to encourage students to see the uniqueness of every client situation and to develop a sense of enquiry about the meaning of their experiences (Wong *et al.* 1997). Glaze (2001a) points out that a curriculum shift has taken place from positivist behavioural paradigms to more qualitative approaches, drawing on emancipatory philosophy and critical social theory, and reflection is seen as a vehicle for the promotion of this. This is also echoed in the development of more facilitative styles of learning in professional education generally, which has been influenced by the work of Friere (1972) and Rogers (1983) among others. It is inevitable that some students are more prepared for this style of education than others due to their past experiences and their independence as learners, as can be seen in some of the research evidence on reflection in nursing in Chapter 1.

Starting with reflection

The students felt that they were already equipped with reflective skills before they started their nursing course. Interestingly, the student below talks about his evident critical thinking ability but is able to distinguish his ability very clearly from his attitude:

'If you interpret reflection as thinking critically then I would say I have always done that... I learnt it as an academic tool here; I learnt to value it in my second year.'

Another student learnt about reflection formally through a counselling course before starting her nursing course, where they used Kolb's learning cycle and were asked to write down what they thought:

'You plod along and then you grow a bit; doing reflection on that counselling course was a big learning curve.'

Structure or no structure?

The students had their own opinions about the use of frameworks for reflection. They saw their value for some people but did not necessarily use them themselves, and this may well reflect their confidence and maturity in using their reflective abilities. There are varying opinions about the use of reflective frameworks (Ghaye & Lilyman 1997; Greenwood 1998; Bulman 2000; Johns 2000), and their use needs to be considered critically. As the student identifies below, they are useful for those seeking some sort of initial guidance but at their worst they can restrict and oppress people's free expression (Bolton 2001):

> 'I think Gibbs' cycle had been introduced to help people who have not even thought about doing reflection before. And I know people who have gone through each part of it but I don't think I've ever done that. I do it more generally; I find it easier not to be so structured.'

Challenging the pursuit of change

The issue of critical reflection being characterised by emancipation and change was something the students spent some time discussing. They challenged the view that change could always be the ultimate goal of critical reflection (Carr & Kemmis 1986), pointing out the realities of practice and their relatively powerless positions as student nurses within the system. This could, I suppose, be interpreted as conforming to the bureaucratic system or equally could be seen as a pragmatic approach, because it is not always possible to change something all of the time. Jarvis and Gibson (1997) urge us not to assume that all reflective learning has to be revolutionary or that it will be automatically innovative. Research studies also suggest that the reflective process may well highlight the inability to change things in practice for people (Duke & Appleton 2000; Graham 2000; Hart *et al.* 2000, Paget 2001). Using their own experiences, students echoed the issues raised by the theorists:

> 'It [reflection-on-action] is expected to be shared through the reflective cycle [Gibbs 1988] and sometimes you can't go through the cycle, sometimes you're right at the point where you say OK I'll change it when I'm a ward manager or when I'm the Prime Minister! I can't always change things; sometimes you get to a point where you say OK I'm just aware of that.'

> 'Nursing is very often seen from the humanistic perspective; you're a lovely nurse; you have a lovely relationship with the patient! A lot of things are structural, political, just society and you can't do anything about that.'

> 'There are many small problems that you can't find an immediate solution to and without reflecting on them you wouldn't even know it was a problem would you?'

> 'We're not in a powerful position (as students) on the wards.'

One student also described talking with a graduate and listening to the account of her disastrous attempts to facilitate change in her clinical area; consequently students felt that developing critical skills was not enough and that being equipped with skills on how to manage change was also important. They were conscious of the cultural, political and organisational issues that affect the ability to change things, and were aware of the limits of education and of themselves. (In Chapter 2 Sue Atkins highlights the need to consider skills for change management.)

Learning and facilitating reflection

The students also had opinions on the learning and facilitation of reflection, commenting on the relevance of life experience and the importance of effective facilitation. They were able to recognise the subtleties involved in getting facilitation right and in encouraging students to develop confidence in reflecting on their experience:

> 'I think the more life experience you've got; the more you've got to base your reflection on. So for the younger students it's possible that it's more difficult to learn to reflect.'

> 'There's a definite difference [in the way people facilitate reflection]; some people have the ability to draw out of you much deeper reflection. I had a link lecturer who used to come onto the ward, she'd just go "Right, what's happened, how did you feel, how did the other person feel?" Just make me think about it on a level I probably wouldn't have done.'

> 'I think I would have liked more challenge and reflection in seminars. If you don't do it with your mentor or link lecturer, there's only your seminar leader, otherwise you're only doing it with your peer group and that's not as challenging sometimes.'

> 'It's hard to challenge without making other people defensive. . .'

> 'You don't want to be aggressive, you want to make people critically think, to challenge them in a positive way. Especially with the first year, first term, I think it is very difficult in seminar leaders' shoes to do that in a positive way. Any kind of positive challenge could be interpreted as "don't talk any more, you said something stupid".'

These comments echo the sentiments expressed by teachers above, and a number of nursing studies exploring reflection-on-action suggest that good facilitation is an important factor in the development of students' reflection, (Shields 1995; Clarke & Graham 1996; Stoddart *et al.* 1996; Paget 2001). Good facilitation appears to be highly valued by students in these studies, especially when difficult or emotional issues were raised (Clarke & Graham 1996). However, generally there is a lack of clarity in the literature about how reflection-on-action can be facilitated effectively (Bolton 2001).

Students also expressed opinions on whether it was possible to teach reflection. This appeared to highlight their values around student-centred learning rather than 'filling students up with information and facts':

> 'Can you teach it? It's debateable; it's like spiritual development, you're ready when you're ready. People can point you in the direction and certain people really inspire you, but can you take 150 people and expect them to come out reflecting at the end of it?'

'I see it as personality building not just reflection. I agree you can't teach reflection, but you can value it in a way. I think this course has valued it.'

They also felt that their course could 'sell' the concept of reflection-on-action better to students:

'You could sell it better maybe, to the younger ones; I just hear them moaning.'

This is particularly pertinent in light of challenges and difficulties with reflecting and writing reflectively reported in studies (Richardson & Maltby 1995; Clarke & Graham 1996; Wallace 1996; Francis *et al.* 1998; Glaze 2001a,b; Platzer *et al.* 2000a,b). These studies suggest that students often express initial difficulties with getting to grips with reflection and what is required of them, but often eventually do appreciate the benefits of it as they develop reflective skills.

Exposing feelings

The students suggested that discussing feelings was not something that was difficult or threatening, and there was also a sense that they were in control of what they were prepared to share with others:

'... sometimes if it is strong emotions, it can be difficult. If you sit on the emotions it's not going to do you much good. It's also good being able to stand back from them and observe what's going on.'

'It's rare that I have strong emotions, I think I wouldn't be happy to share them in front of many people. But on this course it's never happened that I didn't want to share something, because it was such strong emotions that I didn't want to.'

However, despite this assurance, feelings can often affect our learning when we least expect it. One student went on to describe how getting in touch with her feelings through an incident in her practice, helped her to connect with how she felt about patients dying after failed resuscitation attempts. Up until then, she had felt very detached when involved in resuscitation. She commented that learning happened to us all the time and that often we are not able to capture it. In this situation it was her mentor's actions that enabled her to begin to examine her feelings about people not surviving resuscitation:

'My mentor put a flower on her pillow next to her head and I just looked at it and when I went home that night, pow! I was able to be less clinically detached and look at the emotions that I should have felt. It allowed me to become more involved; the trigger was the mentor putting the flower on the pillow. It was a beautiful flower; I said thank you to her the next time, it was a really powerful thing.'

Making a difference to practice

Students felt that reflection made a difference to the way they cared for their patients and readily gave examples of their practical experience to illustrate this. One had reflected on a home visit with an occupational therapist:

'It made me realise how I wasn't helping people in hospital to move towards independence. I might not have reflected on it so deeply, if I hadn't done it for a reflective essay.'

She also described an incident involving a lady who would not take her medication:

'It made me realise how blinking compliant everyone else was! I had real difficulty with this patient for days and days and suddenly I thought, she's trying to teach me something. It challenged me to think about what was going on and made me encourage people not to be so compliant. I tell them what I'm doing, rather than put the pills there; it changed my attitude completely.'

Another student expressed how reflection affected his nursing care in more general ways:

'... I think the major thing with all the personality building, self-awareness, awareness of role, has made me realise that nursing is not just doing the techniques (the medical bits), but all aspects such as talking, listening, social problems, empowering, which are mainly learnt through reflection; I couldn't have learnt them from a textbook. All of that is important in my role as a nurse to critically challenge cultural stereotypes and present practice; to improve it through reflection. Through this training I understand that reflection is valued, I value it and then hopefully other people will value my reflective contribution – if they don't I will do it anyway!'

The importance of theory

Students were clear that linking theory with their practice was important in enabling them to check out their knowledge, maintain their critical ability and broaden their understanding.

A student commenting on reflective writing:

'Getting the theory in as well, is also useful, getting theory in and thinking how I can use it; research, evidence-based practice.'

'There's a lack of specific evidence for some practice so we've been made to be critical about what we do.'

'Reading is seen as academic but to me it is a key part of reflection, it opens up the vast knowledge base out there.'

These ideas are reflected in studies by Glaze (2001a,b) and Wong *et al.* (1997). Participants in Glaze's study raised the importance of theory and literature to reaffirm and explore their ideas and Wong *et al.*'s study also highlights the need for students to integrate literature into their practice experiences in order to broaden and inform their reflection. McKenzie (2002), however, criticises nurses for not allowing their subjective experience to stand alone, seeking established theory to justify and qualify their theories in use. His argument is justified if nurses did not, in reflective style, also evaluate and judge the value and quality of current literature and how it enhances and informs their practice. There is also the possibility that his view may idealise the process of learning from experience; human judgement is not infallible and reflective practitioners would do well to challenge and broaden their thinking through artful coaching, discussion with peers and critical reading.

Conclusion

This chapter has hopefully provided an insight into some of the realities of teaching and learning about reflective practice. Reality of course, can never be fully captured in a book, but hopefully the voices of teachers and students above help to create a picture of the concerns and challenges of some of those teaching and learning about reflection. One respected and experienced colleague confessed to me after a focus group that she wasn't sure that she would have anything useful to say and seemed genuinely surprised by what she was able to contribute. This helped to reassert my belief in uncovering the experiences of those involved in reflective education in order to learn more about how teachers and nurses have interpreted and are using reflection-on-action to teach and learn about nursing. It also brought me back to the notion of 'making the ordinary seem extraordinary' (Atkins & Murphy 1993; Bolton 2001), because there is a need to unpick and examine the ordinary (everyday reflective teaching and learning), so that we can learn something from it.

Acknowledgements

My thanks to Sue Atkins, Enrico Ferrari, Diana Ferguson, Georgie Hawley, Stephanie Hobson, Steph Hodgeson, Jackie Hunt and Charlotte Maddison for agreeing so willingly to share their thoughts and experiences.

References

Atkins, S. & Murphy C. (1993) Reflection: a review of the literature. *Journal of Advanced Nursing*, **18** (8), 1188–92.

Bolton, G. (2001) *Reflective Practice. Writing and Professional Development*. Paul Chapman Publishing Ltd, London.

Bulman, C. (2000) Exemplars of reflection: A chance to learn through the inspiration of others. In: *Reflective Practice in Nursing. The Growth of the Professional Practitioner* (eds S. Burns & C. Bulman).

Bulman, C. & Burns, S. (2000) Students' Perspectives on Reflective Practice. In: *Reflective Practice in Nursing. The Growth of the Professional Practitioner* (eds S. Burns & C. Bulman). Blackwell Science, Oxford.

Carr, W. & Kemmis, S. (1986) *Becoming Critical: Education, Knowledge and Action Research*. The Falmer Press, London.

Clarke, D.J. & Graham, M. (1996) Reflective practice, the use of reflective diaries by experienced registered nurses. *Nursing Review*, **15** (1), 26–9.

Duke, S. (2000) The experience of becoming reflective. In: *Reflective Practice in Nursing: The Growth of the Professional Practitioner*, (eds S. Burns & C. Bulman). Blackwell Science, Oxford.

Duke, S. & Appleton, J. (2000) The use of reflection in a palliative care programme: a quantitative study of reflective skills over an academic year. *Journal of Advanced Nursing,* **32**(6), 1557–68.

Durgahee, T. (1996) Promoting reflection in post-graduate nursing: a theoretical model. *Nurse Education Today,* 16, 419–26.

Fonteyn, M.E. & Cahill, M. (1998) The use of clinical logs to improve nursing students' metacognition: a pilot study. *Journal of Advanced Nursing,* **28**(1), 149–54.

Francis, D., Owens, J. & Tollefson, J. (1998) 'It comes together at the end': the impact of a one-year subject in nursing inquiry on philosophies of nursing. *Nursing Inquiry,* 5, 268–78.

Friere, P. (1972) *Pedagogy of the Oppressed.* Herder and Herder, New York.

Ghaye, Y. & Lilyman, S. (1997) *Learning Journals and Critical Incidents: Reflective Practice for Health Care Professionals.* Quay Books, Mark Allen Publishing Ltd, London.

Gibbs, G. (1988) *Learning by Doing. A Guide to Teaching and Learning Methods.* Oxford Polytechnic, Oxford.

Glaze, J. (2001a) Reflection as a transforming process: student advanced nurse practitioners' experiences on developing reflective skills as part of an MSc programme. *Journal of Advanced Nursing,* **34** (5) 639–47.

Glaze, J. (2001b) Stages in coming to terms with reflection: student advanced nurse practitioners' perceptions of their reflective journeys. *Journal of Advanced Nursing,* **37** (3), 265–72.

Graham, I.W. (2000) Reflective practice and its role in mental health nurses' practice development: a year long study. *Journal of Psychiatric and Mental Health Nursing,* 7, 109–17.

Greenwood, J. (1998) The role of reflection in single and double loop learning. *Journal of Advanced Nursing,* **27** (5), 1048–53.

Hallett, C.E. (1997) Learning through reflection in the community: the relevance of Schön's theories of coaching to nursing education. *International Journal of Nursing Studies,* **34** (2), 103–10.

Hart, G., Clinton, M., Edwards, H., Evans, K., Lunney, P., Posner, N., Tooth, B., Weir, D. & Ryan, Y. (2000) Accelerated professional development and peer consultation: Two strategies for continuing professional education for nurses. *The Journal of Continuing Education in Nursing* **31** (1), 28–37.

Holms, D. & Stephenson, S. (1994) Reflection – A student's perspective. In: *Reflective Practice in Nursing. The Growth of the Professional Practitioner* (eds A. Palmer, S. Burns & C. Bulman).

Honey, P. & Mumford, A. (1986) *The Manual of Learning Styles.* Homey, Maidenhead.

Hyrkas, K., Tarkka, M.T. & Paunonen-Ilmonen, M. (2001) Teacher candidates' reflective teaching and learning in a hospital setting – changing the pattern of practical training: a challenge to growing into teacher hood. *Journal of Advanced Nursing,* **33** (4), 503–11.

Jarvis, P. & Gibson S. (eds) (1997) *The Teacher, Practitioner and Mentor in Nursing, Midwifery, Health Visiting and the Social Services,* 2nd edn. Stanley Thornes, Cheltenham.

Jasper, M.A. (1999) Nurse's perceptions of the value of written reflection. *Nurse Education Today,* 19, 452–63.

Johns, C. (2000) *Becoming a Reflective Practitioner. A reflective and holistic approach to clinical nursing, practice development and clinical supervision.* Blackwell Science, Oxford.

Landeen, J., Byrne, C. & Brown, B. (1995) Exploring the lived experiences of psychiatric nursing students through self-reflective journals. *Journal of Advanced Nursing,* 21, 878–85.

Mallik, M. (1998) The role of nurse educators in the development of reflective practitioners: a selective case study of the Australian and UK experience. *Nurse Education Today,* 18, 52–63.

McCaugherty, D. (1991) The use of a teaching model to promote reflection and the experiential integration of theory and practice in first-year student nurses: an action research project. *Journal of Advanced Nursing*,16, 534–43.

McKenzie, R. (2002) The importance of philosophical congruence for therapeutic use of self in practice. In: *Therapeutic Nursing. Improving Care through Self Awareness and Reflection* (ed. D. Freshwater). Sage Publications, London.

Mountford, B. & Rogers, L. (1996) Using individual and group reflection in and on assessment as a tool for effective learning. *Journal of Advanced Nursing*, 24, 1127–34.

Page, S. & Meerabeau, L. (2000) Achieving change through reflective practice: closing the loop. *Nurse Education Today*, 20, 365–72.

Paget, T. (2001) Reflective practice and clinical outcomes: practitioners' views on how reflective practice has influenced their clinical practice. *Journal of Clinical Nursing*, 10, 204–14.

Platzer, H., Blake, D. & Ashford, D. (2000a) Barriers to learning from reflection: a study of the use of group work with post-registration students. *Journal of Advanced Nursing*, 31 (5), 1001–8.

Platzer, H., Blake, D. & Ashford, D. (2000b) An evaluation of process and outcomes from learning through reflective practice groups on a post-registration nursing course. *Journal of Advanced Nursing*, 31 (3), 689–95.

Richardson, G. & Maltby, H. (1995) Reflection on practice: enhancing student learning. *Journal of Advanced Nursing*, 22, 235–42.

Riley-Doucet, C. & Wilson, S. (1997) A three-step method of self-reflection using reflective journal writing. *Journal of Advanced Nursing*, 25, 964–8.

Rogers, C. (1983) *Freedom to Learn in the 80s.* Merrill, Columbus, Ohio.

Scanlan, J M. & Chernomas, W.M. (1997) Developing the reflective teacher. *Journal of Advanced Nursing*, 25, 1138–43.

Scanlan, J.M., Dean Care, W. & Udod S. (2002) Unraveling the unknowns of reflection in classroom teaching. *Journal of Advanced Nursing*, 38(2), 136–13.

Shields, E. (1995) Reflection and learning in student nurses. *Nurse Education Today*, 15, 452–8.

Spencer, N. & Newell, R. (1999) The use of brief written educational material to promote reflection amongst trained nurses: a pilot study. *Nurse Education Today*, 19, 347–56.

Stoddart, B., Cope, P., Inglis, B., McIntosh, C. & Hislop, S. (1996) Student reflective groups as a Scottish College of Nursing. *Nursing Education Today*, 16, 437–42.

Wallace, D. (1996) Experiential learning and critical thinking in nursing. *Nursing Standard*, 24 (10), 31, 43–7.

Wong, F.K.Y, Loke, A.Y.L., Wong, M., Tse, H., Kan, E. & Kember, D. (1997) An action research study into the development of nurses as reflective practitioners. *Journal of Nursing Education*, 36 (10), 476–81.

Chapter 8

When Reflection Becomes a Cul-de-sac – Strategies to Find the Focus and Move On

Sue Duke

Introduction

In the previous edition of this book, I described my experiences of becoming reflective. Based on the themes from my reflective journals, I tried to illustrate how I moved from 'better have a go' to 'linking thinking and doing'. I argued that my ability to reflect developed over time and contributed to the development of my practice and expertise, enabling me to transfer skills from my clinical practice to my education, research and management practice. Reflection helped me to create a dynamic between thought and action in which such action both recreates my understanding of a situation and transforms the situation. I ended the chapter by saying that I was sure the story I had traced about my experience of reflection would continue to develop 'because reflection has become part of me. It is about who I am as a person and if I have an intention to continue to grow as a person then reflection will always be part of my life'.

Since writing the chapter in the previous edition I have changed my role and am now a nurse consultant in palliative care. In this chapter I describe how reflection has enabled me to make sense of the new challenges that this post has posed – to combine reflective thought and action to establish and develop this role. The main theme of the chapter is how to establish a focus for reflection, to recognise what an experience is about, in order to progress to analysis and action. Despite having experience in reflection and in the elements of the nurse consultant role (expert practice; education; practice and service development; research and evaluation), there was much about my experience as a nurse consultant that I could not identify or name. This often resulted in me being stuck between describing an experience and the feelings related to it and not being able to progress to understanding the experience. I have used various strategies to help me become unstuck; I have continued to use critical friends and my clinical supervisor and through dialogue have come to understand my practice from different perspectives. However, I have also used a variety of analytical strategies to further explore practice in an intentional way and to understand the meaning within my experiences. This chapter focuses on these strategies in the hope that they will help you, if you get stuck in the reflective cycle as I do at times. I have structured the chapter around 'moments' in my experience of developing the role of nurse consultant, chosen to illustrate reflective strategies such as poetry, metaphor and concept mapping. This chapter is a story about how I have used such strategies to broaden and develop my skills in reflection, rather than a coherent story of being a nurse consultant. The chapter ends with an evaluation of such strategies and their applicability to reflection and expert practice.

Bringing the role of nurse consultant alive

'Today I have had the first stabs of fear about what I have done – what is this thing called a nurse consultant? How am I going to bring it to life in a way that is true to my beliefs about the role and about nursing? How I am going to marry all the different expectations that people have of this role and the expected clinical focus with the other dimensions of the role?'

(4 May 2000)

'I went to meet a consultant as part of my orientation. After I had explained what I thought my role was – that I was a consultant like her, that I was a nurse rather than a doctor and that my speciality was palliative care – she was visibly irritated and replied "right, let's see how helpful you might be" and swept me along the corridor to the ward were she was due to do her round. I had not met the nursing team and felt awkward when asked my opinion about someone who had arrested that morning. I was worried that the nurses would feel that I was masking their voice. Afterwards, the consultant said that she would be happy to see me at any of her rounds. Later the unit manager came to see me to express her delight that I made a positive impact on the consultant, that she had been guided by what I said about the palliative care needs of the person we discussed. When I returned to the ward the next day to talk to the nurses about it, they were pleased to have been supported. So what does this all mean with respect to the role of the nurse consultant?'

(19 May 2000)

'Met with the university again today. More dragging of feet about what my role can be. More misunderstandings of why I need this link. More devaluing of my expertise – somehow it is seen that my change of role has lessened my ability to teach, to be involved in curriculum design, and I am being squeezed into a role that is about being an amateur educationalist rather than one that will empower me to facilitate practice education. I am so frustrated.'

(27 July 2000)

'I met with the palliative care consultants. . . I explained my role and emphasised being a nurse and therefore the complementary nature of my role to their's. They asked me what the difference would be between our roles and I discussed my beliefs about nursing and the emphasis on caring. They replied that they cared too and that this was an important part of the speciality: palliative *care*. I felt confused and barren – what am I going to be? How am I going to be in a way that

marks this role as contributory to patient care – let alone distinctive and influential to enhancing patient outcomes?'

(June 2000)

These reflective excerpts are typical of early entries in my reflective journal about
being a nurse consultant. Contrary to the media hype of nurse consultants as
'super nurse' (a *Nursing Times* cartoon character based on Superman), it was
difficult to get a hold on what the role looked like. I had a good theoretical
understanding and a concrete conceptualisation of the role, but I needed to bring it
alive, to live the theory and policy descriptions of the role. Because I was very
excited about this opportunity, for a while I did not address the difficulties that I
was having in forming an identity as a nurse consultant. In effect I was avoiding the
meaning of my journal entries and therefore continuing to experience feelings of
frustration and anxiety. I therefore tried another strategy: rather than trying to
understand my experience through reflective analysis, I played with words that
captured my experience and then organised them to make a coherent summary of
this experience. Richardson (2000, p.933) describes how 'setting words together
in new configurations lets us hear, see and feel the world in new dimensions'. I
tried to capture the meaning of each of the reflective entries cited above in one
word – homeless, lifeless, vacuum, empty. Arranging these words to describe the
experience in the reflection formed the following verse:

Homeless concept,
Empty form,
Spatial vacuum,
Lifeless born.

This expression helped me to understand why it was difficult to bring the role to
life – although I knew about the concept theoretically, there was no practice model
to follow.

Understanding the root of the emotions that I was experiencing enabled me to
analyse the role in a different way. I thought about the two words that construct the
role title – nurse and consultant – and examined journal entries that dwelt on these
concepts. This led to an understanding that some of the tension that I was
experiencing about my identity was matched by the tension between 'consultant'
and 'nurse'. 'Consultant' was by far the most dominant word of my title; people
took notice of me and treated me in the way that I had witnessed medical consultants being treated, whereas I wanted the word 'nurse' to be paramount. I was
concerned that this would subjugate the nursing focus of the role and parallel my
professional experience in which nursing has always struggled to have a voice.

The emphasis on consultant raised other dilemmas. Doctors are socialised into
the role of consultant through their careers and preparation for this post. The role
of nurse consultant is new and therefore nurses have not been socialised into this
role. Socialisation gives people an understanding of what is expected of them. It
shapes our values, thinking frameworks and how we act. I had only experienced
consultant posts through my socialisation as a nurse and this had prepared me to
act as a nurse with respect to consultants, rather than as a consultant. I worried
that I might commit 'professional suicide' unknowingly (do something that was

deemed as being 'unprofessional' for a consultant). My lack of socialisation into that role meant that my understanding about the word consultant was drawn to the stereotypical, for example, to behave in a particular way, such as that described by Elcock (1996) as aloof and elitist, and to do things in a particular way, for example, by assuming leadership (Warelow 1996) and a 'we decide, you carry it out' approach to the division of labour (Colt 1997). I wanted to avoid integrating these stereotypes into my interpretation of a consultant role, but some of the things that were being expected of me reinforced them. For example, in the critical incident that follows there was an expectation that I would focus on pharmacological interventions for someone's pain:

> 'Patient = young women in her 50s, history of breast cancer eight years ago, recently presented with brain metastases, had surgery and radical brain radiotherapy. She was admitted from clinic, as unable to move because of pain.
>
> One day later: hospital Macmillan nurse – "I'm really glad to see you Sue; I want to ask your advice about a patient I saw yesterday." Reviewed the patient and followed through over the next few days – complex pain from bony secondaries and nerve compression from L1-2 and L4-5. Made various suggestions about the management of the pain over the next few days – all accepted and instigated by SHO [Senior House Officer]; pain gradually improved but still severe (although patient now moving around in bed comfortably).
>
> Asked the consultant in palliative medicine to review; she agreed with what I had done and my assessment about where we were – needing to try 4th line neuropathic drugs, e.g. subcutaneous Ketamine. Agreed this would be more safely managed in palliative care unit and arrangements made for transfer – this happened two weeks after admission.'

Although there were many affirming things raised for me in this critical incident – the developing relationship with the Macmillan nurses and being able to complement their skills and knowledge about complicated pain; the opportunities it raised for informal education about neuropathic pain with various nurses, student nurses and the SHO; the reassurance I had about my clinical knowledge and skills – I had several concerns. These included:

- The consultation was predominately focused on how to manage this pain, which was appropriate but only one aspect of this person's experience, albeit that the pain was the predominant experience for this person for much of the time I was involved.
- How to bring a nursing focus to the role of nurse consultant when the things wanted of me are how to manage this pain, which because of its complexity is predominantly through medications – how do I make assessment and support skills explicit when drug management is the predominant focus? How do I ensure adequate psychosocial support for example?
- How do I not fall into a medical model, e.g. leaving support of the patient and family to the nurses on the ward or to the Macmillan nurses and concentrating on assessment and medications?

Other thoughts about this incident:

- Much of my assessment of this person's pain was done by the patient's verbal report, whereas the consultant in palliative medicine examined the patient (e.g. did a neurological examination) – it is tempting to think that this may help my assessment and to therefore carry out examinations myself. Leaving aside the issues about accountability, about my competence to do this; would incorporating examination into my practice reinforce a medical approach? Would this influence how people might view me and therefore use me or would this benefit patient care?

(13 July 2000)

I addressed my concerns about the role of consultant by establishing a critical dialogue with a palliative medicine consultant. I spent three days, spread over a three-month period, observing her practice with a focus on how she behaved towards people and how people behaved towards her. I wrote up these observations and we critically reflected on them in the same way as if we were undertaking a participant ethnographic study. An example of the questions raised from the field notes is given opposite (Table 8.1). The resulting discussion helped me to reconcile the tension between nurse and consultant – it helped me to frame the limits of my role – what I could ask others to legitimately do (for example, that it would be expected for me to ask a SHO to undertake a neurological examination rather than to do it myself) – and where the role of nurse consultant and medical consultant met and diverged (for example, I might undertake an assessment of pain in a very similar way and recommend the same pharmacological strategies but I also help the patient and family to cope with pain through nursing strategies focused on comfort).

Finding a place and being put in my place: where vampires, pirates and aliens roam

Once I understood the tensions between the role of consultant and nurse, I was able to begin to find a place for the role within the organisation. This involved developing relationships with other professionals and managing a delicate balance between 'finding a place' and 'being put in my place'. The attempts to 'put me in my place' were subtle and by themselves nothing very much to note, but they had an intrinsic emotional significance that I found difficult to put into words. Using metaphors helped me to voice these experiences, express them in a way that was safe, and to understand what they were about: the process of controlling access to occupation and status. Three metaphors were involved in this process: vampires, pirates and aliens. I read about these fictional characters first – sensing that there was something about them that captured my experience, but not being sure why. Once I knew more about the typical behaviours of the characters, I was able to link them with my examples from my experience and analyse them, eventually seeing the applicability of sociological theory on occupational closure. A short summary of each now follows.

Vampires are described in the Longman Modern English Dictionary as corpses that come alive at night, fizzle up in the sunshine and drink blood. Humans turn

Table 8.1 Observations and critical questions used for dialogue.

Observation	Questions
Review patient on ward with neuropathic pain Z (palliative medical consultant) reviews notes Looks on board to find out who primary nurse for this patient is Looks for nurse Asks nurse about patient mobilising – is she getting up at all? Nurse says unable to move legs very much, so in bed – radiotherapy is finishing soon and Z wondering whether patient is ready for rehabilitation or what plans might be re discharge Z goes to patient Introduces self and me Z reviews pain Asks questions, prompts, summarises Debates progress of pain management with patient and reviews progress generally Questions centre around site/location of the pain, sensation, intensity, perceived effectiveness of drugs, patterns of pain, perceived progress, and perceived recovery. Some questions around perceived future – Z asking about future and possibilities Patient seems to have very positive aspirations for the future that centre on being totally rehabilitated – i.e. no longer unable to move legs – Z guides this discussion to possibilities that rehab may take time and may not be complete etc. Follow up arrangements discussed with patient: 'one of the team will review you later in the week' Write up suggestions/advice in notes SHO at desk, discussion with SHO re issues raised in conversation with patient – hopes for rehab and her perceptions of what this means SHO did not look up or make eye contact with Z Discusses patient with nurse Leaves ward.	Strikes me that this review is atypical to consultants – i.e. usually have a 'train' of people with them – do you think that this is particular to palliative care, i.e. consultants regularly reviewing patients not as part of a 'ward round'. What do you think the implications of this are sociologically rather than clinically? For example, what does a train of people on a ward round signify? Does this have meaning for a consultant with respect to their credibility or status (for example, one of the oncologists likes me on his round as it boosts his standing – he describes it as 'raising his round'). If so, what does this mean for single conducted rounds like this review? Do you think patients and families will judge status in this way? What were the influences of me observing you on your status as viewed by staff and patients do you think? How does this compare with the lack of interest and courtesy afforded you by the SHO – would she behave like this with the consultant that she is currently working with do you think?

into vampires when bitten, the verb 'to turn' describing this process. Vampires describe the negotiation involved in bringing the concept of nurse consultant alive collaboratively rather than competitively. I have encountered tests of whether I can 'stand the heat' through challenges that assess my knowledge and analytical skills, and I am goaded to draw blood by seeing whether I will return insults or put up a fight.

Pirates are to do with working outside the rules, trespassing, plundering treasure. They are often depicted as heroes rather than as villains, but they need to earn this status. They describe the negotiation of place in the organisation. For example, I have needed to address the perception that I am a trespasser who plunders other people's treasure, for example having access to consultant status that belongs to medicine without having done the work or made the sacrifices to deserve this status (learned the ropes) or as a threat to the status of clinical nurse specialists. This has been offset by demonstrating that I have credibility and can offer treasure, often requested by the phrase: 'Sue can I pick your brains'. On rare occasions pirates fly a red flag (Jolly Roger) which signals 'take no quarter' (no survivors). I recognise red Jolly Rogers by the fight or rage invoked within me. For example, I hoisted a red Jolly Roger in response to one hoisted by a medical consultant who asked me to be just a 'pink and fluffy' nurse and to 'forget all that advanced nursing stuff'. On discussing this exchange, he admitted he had been looking for something that would raise such a response in me, because he wanted to understand what was important to me (in this case my values about nursing and the knowledge that underpins it). Such interactions are about negotiating boundaries or territories.

Aliens signify the experience of being a stranger, to a Trust and palliative care service that is new to me, to the role of nurse consultant, to other disciplines. It is about trying to understand different cultures, and the beliefs and values, architecture and thinking schemas that shape these cultures, in order to negotiate my role and its place within it.

I constructed the following poem to order and express these metaphors and this helped to develop a focus for the reflection through creating a concise summary of the experience.

Vampires suck my blood
And wait for me to turn
Like them, competitive.
I strive to stay alive,
And resist the fanged club,
Instead, collaborate.

Pirates treat me as role
Contender, trespasser,
Accuse me of plunder.
I am no skills thief, but
See red Jolly Rogers
Warning, Hold no quarter!

Aliens baffle me
Their culture quite unique.
We find a meeting space
In which to hold debate,
Tentatively touch it,
Learn to communicate.

The sociologists
Tell me these three villains,
Have other names instead.
Tell how professionals
Keep strangers out, double
Closure I read about.

The dangers of these foes
Include demarcation
And peer separation,
Designed to increase power
And increase influence,
Instead makes enemies.

Vampires, pirates, aliens,
Symbolic experience.
Remind me to value
The nurse in consultancy.
Warns me not to oppress
Others or indoctrinate.

The metaphors gave me a safe way to discuss what I was trying to achieve and to express the emotion related to being 'put in my place' without feeling that I was criticising the colleagues involved. Richardson (2000) argues that metaphors enable the experiencing and understanding of one thing in terms of another through comparison. My colleagues recognised the characters of vampires, pirates and aliens because they were both familiar with these as storybook characters and with the characteristics of medical and organisational culture depicted. This enabled them to understand the experience being portrayed but because a comparison was being drawn, they did not have to necessarily identify themselves as those characters or as having the characteristics described. The emotion of the experience was deflected by the metaphor and therefore reduced the potential criticism of the poetry.

Froggatt (1998) describes how metaphors are a practical strategy used by nurses for managing the emotional aspects of their work. She argues that this is necessary because nurses are expected to exercise a degree of control over their emotions. This may explain why I could not fully articulate how I felt about the experiences from which the poem was constructed – I was subject to the norms of emotions and trying to present myself as a nurse consultant in a way that would be true to the expectations inherent in being a nurse and in being experienced (in this instance, able to control my emotions).

In addition to reflecting reality, Froggatt (1998) describes metaphor as a creative force that creates reality. From a qualitative study exploring the sources and function of metaphor in relation to death, dying and bereavement, Spall *et al.* (2001) found that metaphor facilitated the exploration, expression and explanation of difficult situations from a personal perspective. In this way metaphor gave me a way not just to express the emotion related to the experience but to understand what it was related to. I refined this understanding by constructing a poem using the metaphors and my analysis.

The poetic form created a confined space for the expression of the things that I had been exploring. This confined space gave safety for the expression of the emotion related to the metaphors and may explain the more personal nature of the last verse. It also challenged me to be concise and succinct in what I wanted to say and yet gave me the freedom to express something that 'rings true' rather than claims to 'be true' (Brady 2000, p.958).

Thus, the combination of poetry and metaphor in the poem achieves a safe way of telling a story about doctors and nurses that does not depend on the stereotypical images. This shifts the moral of the story from what is right or wrong (who should be 'in charge') to what an experience has been like. Carson (1998, p.233) summarises this as: 'something that both "figures" in the light of our understanding of what life is generally like and throws light on the road we've travelled'. Such a shift also enabled an alternative analysis of the experience. As the common frameworks of reflection suggest, once an experience is described and the feelings related to that experience attended to, different perspectives can be explored and assumptions challenged. Being free of the emotion helped me check my assumption that most interactions were characterised by this experience. I found that many were not and therefore could look towards alternative explanations for the experience. My analysis shifted from occupational closure, in effect a stereotypical analysis, towards understanding changes in the socio-cultural context. Occupational closure stresses knowledge as the key to power base, whereas knowledge is increasingly contested because of the increasing access to information (Delanty 1999). In this context knowledge and expertise are open to question and judgement, through what Delanty (1999) calls discursive regulation by 'reflexive and self-regulating individuals'. This thinking raised a new perspective of my role that was about having a place that fitted with what I was doing at any one moment. It changed my search for a distinctive role to one that recognised the importance of flexibility, and in turn this paradoxically enhanced my credibility, because I was able to demonstrate a broader range of skills and expose my vulnerability.

Whose voice is being heard and scanning the noise

One of the other issues of context that I have been struggling with is the dynamic between the environment of the acute hospital and palliative care and how I negotiate the philosophies inherent within these two things. In some sense this is about whose voice is being heard and how as a nurse, I can help people to have a voice. Practice is often about competing voices, this causing a noise through which no one can be heard clearly. One of the key things about a nurse's role in this noise is to create an environment that can act as a filter to metaphorically turn down the volume of some voices, in order that others are heard. For example, breaking bad news on an acute ward where a patient cannot be moved into a quiet space results in this news competing with other conversations. I see my role as a nurse in these situations being pivotal to creating a space in which the patient can concentrate on what is being said, rather than being distracted by the 'surround sound'. I do this by reshaping the space around the bed, ensuring that the teller of the bad news feels supported so that she or he can concentrate on the patient rather than on what they are going to say, ensuring that the patient feels supported by including and welcoming into this space people important to them. I try and prepare patients for such conversations by listening to their concerns beforehand, and helping them to rehearse the questions they might want to ask. Portraying the challenge of this practice in discussion is difficult because discussion is constructed in a clear and logical way, whereas practice is messy, ambiguous and fragmented. Discussion can also make practice seem abstract and disembodied (Gadow 2000).

Since my role is not just about supporting patients and their families, and includes teaching others about practice, I have to find ways of transforming the messiness and ambiguous reality of practice into something that can be understood by those I am teaching. In discussing how to bring practice alive, Gadow (2000) describes the use of a poetic form called motet. Motets are choral works, usually unaccompanied, of sacred Latin texts. They were popular from the thirteenth to sixteenth centuries. In this form different parts of the text are sung simultaneously and illuminate the different voices or perspectives involved in a situation. Gadow argues that 'the differing, even opposing, narratives of the several voices, ends expectations of unity and of certainty. The voices interrupt each other, each one affecting the sound of the others. A listener follows one and then another without being able to hear them individually or all at once' (p.95).

Figure 8.1 is an attempt to use motet to illustrate the context surrounding a patient being told bad news. It shows all the voices that were going on around her that I was trying to quieten by creating a space in which she could hear what she was being told. To me, this 'score' brings alive the challenges of creating a space, because it makes explicit the noise that is present and the salience of some of this noise to me – I was listening in on these conversations while concentrating on the patient and her family and the doctor telling her the news, because these other conversations are telling me something about the health of the other patients nearby and the personality and skill of the nurses caring for them. I was filtering the conversations for cues that would alert me to things I needed to attend to: Was the patient in the opposite bed less distressed now? Did the clinical nurse specialist talking to her need some support after being shouted at? Was the patient in the next bed being coerced into being admitted into a hospice? Were the 'proper' checks done when the blood was put up? Was the nurse's comment, 'good', patronising or part of a rich exchange between the patient and nurse that reassured her about the transfusion?

Not walking the talk

The last moment of being a nurse consultant that I want to describe is related to my attempts to integrate clinical and educational practice. I described in the previous edition of this book how I began my journey as a reflective practitioner by setting some students an assignment that involved reflection, and how I began to keep a reflective journal as a result of this – that it did not seem right to ask students to do

1. Patient being told the cancer has progressed and that emergency treatment is needed to stop it pressing on her spinal cord and causing paralysis. Doctor's voice, very steady and gentle.	. . . yes, the cancer has spread and is in some of the bones in your spine. This is very serious as it can cause paralysis. *Yes, I understand.* We need to start some urgent treatment, some radiotherapy to shrink the cancer to prevent this.
2. Discussion by the opposite bed, specialist nurse discussing hygiene with a patient with a Hickman line. This line has become infected and puts the patient at risk of septicaemia. Patient's voice loud and anguished, nurse's voice begins conversational but becomes defensive.	bath or a shower? WHEN YOU SAY THAT YOU MAKE ME FEEL DIRTY, REALLY DIRTY I'm sorry but I need to know how to help you prevent infection in your line. BUT THAT MAKES ME THINK THAT YOU THINK I AM DIRTY. I'm sorry, I didn't mean to upset you.

3. Nurse with patient in the bed to the left going through safety checks before administering blood. Nurse's voice instrumental but warm.	Can you tell me your name and date of birth?
	      POLLY SMITH 1.2.33.
	      Very good, now you can have your blood.

4. Family with patient in the bed to the right discussing her planned discharge to a hospice after the weekend. Relative's voice reassuring and relieved (that care has been organised). Patient's voice resigned and frightened (that she is ill enough to be needing such care).	So you are going to the hospice?
	      Yes, the nurse sorted it out.
	      Ah! That's nice, Mrs McNally died there, she thought it was a wonderful place, they made her ever so comfortable.
	
	I don't know why I can't go home.
	
	They will look after you.
	But I can look after myself when I get better.

Fig. 8.1 Motet 'Breaking bad news'.

something that I did not do. This 'do what you teach and teach what you do' approach to clinical and education practice has been an important mantra within my nurse consultant role, as it was within my lecturer practitioner role. A concept map (the linking together in diagrammatic form of related ideas) that I drew of my practice as a mentor shattered my complacency about my ability to achieve this integration. I drew the map as a way of trying to understand why I felt that I had not done a very good job as a mentor. The map helped me to see that I had not linked clinical or subject knowledge with the development of education knowledge and had limited the student's learning opportunities as a result and reinforced the separateness of clinical practice and education.

Concept maps used in this way differ from their use as a way to plan an essay or a teaching session. The intention is to use the map to plot thinking in action and by doing this to elicit practical or aesthetic knowledge. For example, a qualitative study by Meijer *et al.* (2002) found that concept maps enabled the decision-making processes and the tacit knowing underpinning practice to be illustrated and debated, and that this tool was well evaluated by students and their mentors. What is interesting in relation to my experience of using a concept map is how it illuminated something that I was not expecting, in a similar way to how the maps in the study by Meijer *et al.* illustrated things that were not being emphasised as important to practice.

There are a couple of things that have come from my experience of using concept maps in this way. The first is related to the expression of thinking in action captured by the map. I find that because I have expertise in several aspects of my role it is easy to be drawn into thinking 'on the hop'. The multiple expectations and functions expected within the nurse consultant role make working life crowded. Often there is little time to think between doing one thing and another and often I am expected to be able to think about several things at once. For short periods this is fine, but when the pressure of work creates a situation where this is expected over long periods then the quality of my work suffers from a lack of reflection. The concept map makes this thinking 'on the hop' explicit and in doing so also makes explicit what was not thought about and consequently what I might have done better if I had created some time for reflection between actions. It is not always easy to reconcile what was with what might have been, and this gives a different essence to reflection that leads to new learning, something that is often enlightening and exciting. In contrast, this experience is much more humbling. It is about reminding myself that however experienced I am, reflection is not just important but essential to acting in the most appropriate way. It reminds me that expertise or the nurse consultant role does not bring infallibility

The second thing is related to the potential for concept maps to elicit artistic knowledge. Such knowledge is shaped by the values we place on things and the way that we think and perceive things. Concept maps therefore bring alive the congruency between how you acted and what you value. In the example I described above, the concept map showed how I was not congruent with the value of 'walking the talk' and some of the possible reasons why this had happened. I had not been aware of this incongruency when I was being a mentor but they were present and therefore would have been noticed by the person I was mentoring. Understanding this helped me to make sense of the feeling that I had not done a good job. The reality was that indeed I had not done a good job. The feelings that this evoked – sadness, shock, frustration with myself – helped me to understand that my value, 'to walk the talk', was still very important to me. This process let me move on to analyse the consequences of what had happened and plan how I will try things out in the future, and to understand the complexities of undertaking the practice education focus of the nurse consultant role.

Reflective strategies – breaking a reflective short circuit

This chapter has described several reflective strategies that have helped me make sense of my experience as a nurse consultant. These strategies are integral to reflection because they enable the process of reflection. What has been interesting

Table 8.2   The role of reflective strategies in progressing reflection.

'Moment' described	Strategy	What this strategy achieved	Reflective facilitated
Bring the role of nurse consultant alive	One word to express the meaning of reflective journal entries, assembled to describe early experience of being a nurse consultant	Recognition and understanding of the negative feelings associated with the role. Identification of a focus for reflective analysis – how to bring the role alive in a way that would celebrate nursing	Analysis of the tension between the words nurse and consultant.
	Ethnographic observation and analysis of the role of consultant	Shifted focus from how to avoid stereotypical attributes of consultant to how to embrace aspects of consultancy that might enable the role of nurse consultant to come to life	Reconcilitation of the tension between the words consultant and nurse. Understanding of the expectations of consultants. Mitigated my fear of committing cultural suicide
			Analysis of the limits of my role, what I can legitimately ask others to do, what I can legitimately do for myself
			Analysis of where the nurse and medical consultant posts met and diverged
Finding a place versus being put in my place	Metaphor and poetry	Legitimised emotions related to establishing a role and identified issues that provoked these emotions	Analysis of role and actions through sociological theory
		Enabled a shift in focus from occupational closure to contested knowledge	Valuing of diversity and flexibility

Contd.

Table 8.2   Contd.

'Moment' described	Strategy	What this strategy achieved	Reflective facilitated
Whose voice is being heard and scanning the noise	Motet	Focus for reflection on context shifted from putting up with the difficulties to how to shape the context and capitalise on the knowledge that the context gives me	Analysis of nursing skills in shaping context and how knowledge embedded in this context is known
Not walking the talk	Concept map	Focus on the root of my feelings in relation to a practice event – incongruence between professing to 'walk the talk' and achieving this	Analysis of the consequences of treating education and subject knowledge as separate

about my experience of reflecting on the role of being a nurse consultant is that despite having experience of and understanding the process of reflection, I have often become stuck between describing a situation and progressing to the analysis. I describe this to the students that I teach as playing ping-pong ball with the description and feelings part of the reflective cycle, a sort of reverberating short circuit. What the strategies have done is enable me to break this short circuit and to highlight the importance of understanding the focus in the reflective description (see Table 8.2). This last point is particularly interesting to me. Although several authors emphasise the focus as an integral part of the reflective process   for example, Benner (1984) and Smith and Russell (1991) discuss the importance of identifying the salience or what was most demanding about the situation – many frameworks of reflection dash over this and progress from description to feelings. Because the role of nurse consultant is a new one, there is little knowledge about it and therefore it has often been difficult to identify a focus. The strategies that I have described like metaphor and poetry have helped me to understand what the salience is, to ask the question that Day (1985, 1993) poses: 'What does the description mean?'

Conclusion: reflection and the expert practitioner

Reflection is a great leveller. It teaches you that, however experienced you are, you still have things to learn. My experience of using reflection to help me make sense of being a nurse consultant has taught me that although I believe myself to be reflective, I am still capable of getting stuck, of playing a metaphorical game of ping-pong ball in the reflective cycle. I have happened across the strategies that I have used to break this short circuit. They raise all sorts of questions for me like 'how can I be so arrogant as to think that I can write poetry when I know so little about this art form?' They shock me with what is revealed, show me the assumptions that I am making in my practice, what I am hiding from myself, how I am being incongruent to my values, how my values need to change. They remind me of what it is like to first find out about the power of reflection – the excitement and compelling nature of understanding something new or afresh, the richness of coming to know yourself. This experience has also taught me that it is important to pay attention to the processes involved in reflection. I have got stuck sometimes, because I have been too impatient to get to the analysis part of the reflective process or because I could not see what the focus of the analysis should be. Time spent sorting out these things is well spent and important in attaining richness and depth to the reflective analysis and to any action that follows.

References

Benner, P. (1984) *From Novice to Expert: Excellence and Power in Clinical Nursing Practice*. Addison-Wesley, Boston.

Brady, L. (2000) Anthropological poetics. In: *Handbook of Qualitative Research* (eds N.K. Denzin & Y.S. Lincoln), 2nd edn, pp.949–80. Sage, London.

Carson, R.A. (1998) The moral of the story. In: *Stories and their Limits* (ed. H.L. Nelson), pp.232–7. Routledge, London.

Colt, C. (1997) 'We decide, you carry it out': a social network analysis of multidisciplinary long-term care teams. *Social Science and Medicine*, 45(9), 1411–21.

Day, C. (1985) Professional learning and researcher intervention. *British Educational Research Journal*, 11(2), 133–51.

Day, C. (1993) Reflection: a necessary but not sufficient condition for professional development. *British Educational Research Journal*, 19(1), 83–93.

Delanty, G. (1999) *Social Theory in a Changing World*. Polity, Cambridge.

Elcock, K. (1996) Focus on specialist nursing. Consultant nurse: an appropriate title for the advanced practitioner? *British Journal of Nursing*, 5(22), 1376–81.

Froggatt, K. (1998) The place of metaphor and language in exploring nurses' emotional work. *Journal of Advanced Nursing*, 28(2), 332–8.

Gadow, S. (2000) Philosophy as falling: aiming for grace. *Nursing Philosophy*, 1, 89–97.

Meijer, P.C., Zanting, A. & Verloop, N. (2002) How can student teachers elicit experienced teachers' practical knowledge? Tools, suggestions and significance. *Journal of Teacher Education*, 53(5), 406–19.

Richardson, L. (2000) Writing a method of inquiry. In: *Handbook of Qualitative Research* (eds N.K. Denzin & Y.S. Lincoln) 2nd edn, pp.923–48. Sage, London.

Smith, A. & Russell, J. (1991) Using critical incidents in nurse education. *Nurse Education Today*, 11(4), 284–91.

Spall, B., Read, S. & Chantry, D. (2001) Metaphor: exploring its origins and therapeutic use in death, dying and bereavement. *International Journal of Palliative Nursing*, 7(7), 345–53.

Warelow, P.J. (1996) Nurse-doctor relationships in multidisciplinary teams: ideal or real? *International Journal of Nursing Practice*, 2(1), 33–9.

Chapter 9
Help to Get You Started – Reflecting on Your Experiences

Chris Bulman

Introduction

It must be pretty evident to you by now that reflection is not easy and that evidence and experience show that time, recall, ethics, emotions and privacy are just some of the issues that need to be thoughtfully considered (Newell 1992; Hargreaves 1997; Mackintosh 1998; Burton 2000). Therefore the experience of using reflection and facilitating its use in students and colleagues, tells me that most people are relieved to be offered some help to get them going. There is no doubt in my mind that looking at other people's reflective writing and being given a few handy hints can boost people's confidence with the whole thing. Also, artful teachers recognise the need to support students in new ways of thinking and learning about their practice, but also realise that critically reflecting on your practice is not an easy journey. Thus here is a final chapter offering exemplars of other people's practice to help you to get started, hopefully complementing other chapters in the book.

Why bother to reflect at all?

If human beings did not possess the ability to be thoughtful about the problems of life, one could question whether we would ever have harnessed the benefits of fire or invented the wheel. Cynics among you will no doubt declare at this point that the trouble with human beings is that we don't do enough developing or learning from our capacity to think.

It is at this stage that the ability to reflect rather than simply be thoughtful is worth dwelling on. Jarvis (1992) suggests that reflection is not just thoughtful practice but a learning experience. Like life, nursing involves situations that are complex and if we are to understand nursing and ourselves as nurses, we need to try and make sense of the complexity (Heath 1998). Wong *et al.* (1997, p.476) suggest that in the real world of practice every nurse–client encounter is unique and there are not always fixed solutions to problems. Consequently, they believe that nurses need to review their repertoire of clinical experience and knowledge before they can suggest innovative ways of 'dealing with complex clinical riddles'.

The trouble with nursing and the complexities of thinking about practice

So the trouble with nursing, as with life in general, is that it is dynamic, constantly changing, challenging, frustrating and exciting often all at the same time. Therefore, as practitioners of nursing it is impossible to declare that we have nursing 'in the bag'; that we know all there is to know or that we have reached a final understanding of practice. In order to develop our understanding of practice we require what Dewey (1933) and Eraut (1994) would refer to as intellectual effort in order to push ourselves further in our inquiry and inquisitiveness about reality. This does, however, have an element of dualism about it, so perhaps what we should talk about is the need for reflective effort which incorporates thinking, feeling and action effort. With reflective effort it is logically also possible that theory development arising from practice could emerge as nurses acquire a more reflective way of practising nursing, giving them the insight to 'grow' nursing theory from practice itself.

It is possible then, with some effort, to explore ourselves as professionals, by reflecting on our experiences, in order to develop our self-awareness and ability to self-evaluate. I think Sue Duke's chapter (Chapter 8) is a wonderful example of that. Importantly, Bolton (2001) points out that we do not practise with one part of ourselves and live our personal lives with the other, so there is certainly some relevance in thinking about the investment in self as part of professional development.

The reflective approach is typified by growth and learning rather than the reliance on ritual and automatic pilot to get us through the day (Schön 1983, 1987; Saylor 1990; Street 1991; Ghaye & Lilyman 1997; Brockbank & McGill 1998; Rolfe *et al.* 2001). Indeed, Jarvis (1992) strongly advocates the need for reflective practice since nurses are dealing with people who, because of their individual nature, require us to be responsive and reflective, instead of simply carrying out routine, ritual and presumption. Reflection also requires a wholehearted approach, as Ghaye and Lilyman (2000, p.97) point out:

> 'It is not something to be 'bolted- on' to courses and programmes of study. We do not believe you can profess to be a reflective practitioner for one day a week and some kind of health care worker for the rest. It is not something that you can commodify; just pick up and put down, buy into or not, almost at will.'

Reflective effort and change

In order to be effective in practice there is a requirement to be purposeful and goal-directed (Street 1991); thus critical reflection cannot just be concerned with understanding, but must also include locating practice within its social and political structures (Bolton 2001) and in changing practice (Driscoll 1994). Achieving this reflective education needs the right culture, one that is conducive to open inquiry, support and challenge, based on practice, with theory related to practice (Goodman 1984). This of course operates on the assumption that people want to strive to change and are not content with benign paternalism, and may give the impression that small considerations and developments in practice are not enough. As Jarvis and Gibson (1997) comment, because of Friere's (1972) work it might be assumed that all reflective learning has to be revolutionary; we must not assume this, or that reflective learning will be automatically innovative. It is also interesting to consider whether encouraging individuals to develop reflection is one way to divert the responsibility for practice away from organisations and entirely on to the wonderfully broad shoulders of practitioners. Cynicism aside, you will certainly be able to detect personal considerations of change and development in the exemplars that follow; however it is always valuable to consider some of these issues in true reflective style.

Another word of caution is justified at this point. I believe that reflection could offer most of us a route toward exploring our ability to be therapeutic in our practice. This can only be achieved by the fostering of self-awareness and an ability to be constructively critical in order to facilitate positive change. We may pay a price for this, however, even though it could be one that is worthwhile in the long run, since reflection is not always comfortable (Saylor 1990; Carr 1996). This is a point amply illustrated in the exemplars that follow. Reflection forces you to face incongruity and uncomfortable facts about nursing, the health services you work in and yourself. You need to consider both the positive and negative aspects before embarking on a reflective pathway, and educationalists introducing reflection as part of a curriculum need to be aware of this too and carefully consider the support required for such an approach (James & Clarke 1994).

Below I have summarised the important issues that arise from the discussion above and it is these that I hope you will be able to identify throughout the exemplars in the rest of the chapter:

- To appreciate that situations in nursing can be complex
- To resolve to try and understand what nursing is about
- To strive to be self-aware and to self-evaluate
- To question routine, ritualisation and the 'taken for granted'
- To develop and challenge current practice.

Helping you to start

Many of the tips mentioned below will seem familiar, as they will have been covered in different contexts throughout the book. They are summarised here to give you the chance to consider what you need to work on at a glance, rather than necessarily ploughing through the book, except where you may require further detail.

The following are worth considering.

Using a framework to help you to reflect

You will find different types of frameworks below that are illustrative of the type of tools that qualified and unqualified nurses have used in order to help them with their reflection, and that have been employed by educationalists and researchers alike to qualify reflection. Take time to have a look at these, noting the critique of them, and think about what might work for you.

Finding someone to reflect with

A colleague, mentor or supervisor can provide a sounding board, open up different perspectives and provide support and guidance. It is helpful to find someone who already has experience of using reflection and who is someone that you trust, if you are going to share and explore your experiences and feelings. The coaching and facilitation role cannot be ignored in the reflective process since it is very easy to slip into non-critical self-affirmation without it. Take a look at Chapter 4 to help you think about this further.

Keeping a reflective journal or diary

Keeping a regular diary is an extremely useful tip, since the memory of events can fade quickly, even for those with the most photographic of memories. You may find it helpful to build up a personal repertoire of experience in your diary, which you will be able to use to reflect back on and draw from, as you gain in experience. Chapter 5 is well worth dwelling on with respect to writing reflectively, and you will also find some useful tips in Chapter 3 on diaries and journals.

Reading the literature

We hope that this whole book will provide you with some useful background on reflection; however, in generous academic spirit there are also some other recent books that you will find helpful: John's latest work (2000), Ghaye and Lilyman's books (1997, 2000), Bolton's (2001) work has particularly caught the imagination of educationalists, and Brockbank and McGills's (1998) book is another useful resource for teachers. A critical look at the wealth of discussion articles about reflection is also worthwhile since it will help you to focus on the pros and cons surrounding reflection. Here are just a few that span from the mid 1980s to early 2000s and offer a variety of views: Clarke (1986); Jarvis (1992); Atkins & Murphy (1993); Day (1993); Greenwood (1993a,b, 1998); Reid (1993); James & Clarke (1994); Richardson (1995); Scanlan & Chernomas (1997); Clinton (1998); Heath (1998); Mallik (1998); Kim (1999); Cotton (2001).

Basically though, it is important that you understand the concepts involved and have a clear idea of what you might personally find helpful in starting to reflect. In Chapter 2 Sue Atkins provides some useful tips and theoretical background on the attributes necessary for true reflection, and Chapter 1 explores some of the latest nursing research on reflection. Additionally, Chapter 7 provides some useful insights into students 'and teachers' perspectives.

Having the courage to change and/or challenge

As mentioned previously, reflection can be painful as well as enlightening, often bringing things to conscious thought that need to be dealt with. However, as old tutor of mine once said, 'If you're finding something uncomfortable it p means you're learning something useful.' This is not always easy to deal with, however, and it benefits from the good support of a mentor/supervisor. Importantly, Hargreaves (1997) warns of the potential vulnerability of students exposed to reflection and advocates the need for support and ethical direction from educationalists. Of course, it is helpful if you work in an environment where positive change and constructive challenge are welcomed in the workplace; it is easier then to be brave and voice your reflections on practice (Cullingford 1991). If you are not in such a position you need to seek out supportive and facilitative networks, before you set off on a reflective pathway.

Some useful frameworks for reflection

Although you may be filled with enthusiasm to begin to reflect, the dilemma of where to start is common. Consequently, I have included some suggestions below for use as frameworks to help with going about the business of reflection. It may be that you feel comfortable with one particular framework and opt to use it every time you reflect. However, it is not essential to use a framework; some practitioners choose not to.

It is also worth remembering Johns' (2000) caution that frameworks or models are just devices to help you with reflection; they are not designed to impose a prescription of what reflection is. Bolton (2001) makes the point that frameworks could be as much about control as guidance, and therefore they should be viewed and used with these critiques in mind. Greenwood (1998) critiquing the work of Argyris and Schön (1974) also comments on the lack of 'double loop learning' potential in some of these frameworks, i.e. they fail to encourage the user to search for alternative actions to achieve the same ends, or to examine the appropriateness or propriety of chosen ends; she believes that they do not encourage critical reflection. She does, however, overlook the fact that frameworks are not the only thing guiding someone's reflection, and while some may not overtly promote a critical theory approach, they do at least guide the user to think about critiquing experience for future action and looking at the influences and consequences of action.

The suggestions below are not exhaustive. There are many more available in the literature; for example, the work of Van Manen (1977), Boud *et al.* (1985), Burnard (1991), Driscoll (1994), Ghaye and Lilyman (1997) and Jay and Johnson (2002), all provide help for the reflective practitioner.

The reflective cycle (Gibbs 1988)

Since reflection is not a static process but a dynamic one, it is appropriate to include a framework with an overt cyclical approach. The reflective framework illustrated in Fig. 9.1 is adapted from a framework for experiential learning and guides you through a series of questions in order to provide structure when reflecting on an experience. You can begin at the top of the cycle asking the

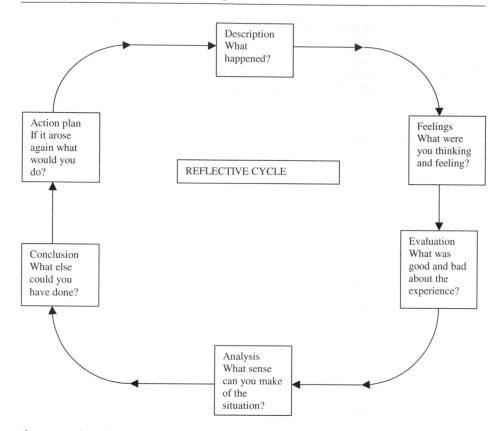

Fig. 9.1   The reflective cycle (Gibbs 1988).

question 'what happened?', and then progress around the cycle in order to explore an experience in practice and to guide the reflective process, and then of course begin all over again by taking a plan for action back into practice and reflecting on your changes. Reid (1993) suggests using Gibbs' cycle in conjunction with Goodman's (1984) levels of reflection; this is useful in order to challenge you to think more critically about the quality of your reflection. Additionally, you do need to accept that the questions in the cycle are pretty broad and that you will need to reflexively consider *your* effect and influence on practice; despite these issues a lot of practitioners like the simplicity of this framework.

Johns' model of structured reflection (Table 9.1) is composed of a series of questions helping the reflective practitioner to tune into an experience and provide structure and meaning to the process of reflection. He has developed this model for structured reflection over several years, realising the usefulness of such a technique, at least in the early stages, to guide people while they get going with reflection. The model has emerged through Chris Johns' extensive work through which practitioners have explored their experiences in supervision, (Johns 1993, 1994, 1995a,b, 2000; Johns & Freshwater 1998). This later version also includes an element of reflexivity which encourages the experienced practitioner particu-

Table 9.1   A Model of Structured Reflection. Adapted from Johns (2000 p47).

Looking in
Find a space to focus on self
Pay attention to your thoughts and emotions
Write down those thoughts and emotions that seem significant in realising desirable work

Looking out
Write a description of the situation surrounding your thoughts and feelings
What issues seem significant?

Aesthetics:	What was I trying to achieve?
	Why did I respond as I did?
	What were the consequences of that for the patient/others/myself?
	How were others feeling?
	How did I know this?
Personal:	Why did I feel the way I did in this situation?
Ethics:	Did I act for the best?
	What factors were influencing me? (Within me or in the environment?)
Empirics:	What knowledge did or should have informed me?
Reflexivity:	Does this connect with previous experiences?
	How could I handle this situation better?
	What would be the consequences of alternative actions for the patient/others/myself?
	How do I *now* feel about this experience?
	Can I support myself and others better as a consequence?
	How available am I to work with patients/families and staff to help them meet their needs?

larly to continue to employ reflective effort in tackling a particular practice issue; this is less evident in other frameworks and is a useful inclusion.

Finally, I have chosen another framework which poses a series of questions for you to work through: Stephenson's reflective framework (Table 9.2). It emerged from the student experiences of Sarah Stephenson, who wrote in the first edition of this book. She was immersed in reflection throughout her pre-registration, undergraduate studies, and her framework is worth sharing with others. I have used Stephenson's framework particularly with students reflecting on their clinical experiences and they have found it a useful and challenging guide to reflective tutorial groups, and so have I.

Frameworks utilising levels of reflection

Theorists have developed work on levels of reflection which has been used by both researchers and educationalists in an attempt to try and qualify people's reflection. It has particular significance in the development of critical reflection and consequently the ability of students to develop and change. A closer look at Mesirow's (1981) and Goodman's (1984) work is useful for both nurses and teachers in identifying some of the attributes that theorists have attached to reflection. This work is of course open to the criticism that reflection can be reduced to levels; however to the pragmatist it offers some pointers in determining what the focus of reflection is about.

Table 9.2   A reflective framework (Stephenson 2000).

Choose a situation from your placement; ask yourself …
• What was my role in this situation?
• Did I feel comfortable or uncomfortable? Why?
• What actions did I take?
• How did I and others act?
• Was it appropriate?
• How could I have improved the situation for myself, the patient, my mentor?
• What can I change in future?
• Do I feel as if I have learnt anything new about myself?
• Did I expect anything different to happen? What and why?
• Has it changed my way of thinking in any way?
• What knowledge from theory and research can I apply to this situation?
• What broader issues, for example ethical, political or social, arise from this situation?
• What do I think about these broader issues?

Mesirow's levels of reflection

Mesirow's (1981) work is influenced by the work of the critical theorist Habermas. Mesirow suggested that adults are capable of being consciously critical or critically reflective and emphasised the importance of self-directed learning. He identified two paths to what he calls perspective transformation or sudden insight into one's assumptions, and transitional movement leading to a revision of those assumptions; he suggested that transformation is perhaps the more common of the two. Importantly Mesirow's work identifies the difficulties and problems of consciousness-raising that Friere (1972) does not highlight in his work. Mesirow suggests that issues such as difficult negotiation and compromise, stalling, backsliding, self-deception and failure are common features – enough to frighten any enthusiastic teacher or student in their bid to improve reflection.

Mesirow's levels of reflectivity (Table 9.3) which derive from his collaborative research work on women college returners and their perspective transformations, have captured the interest of both researchers and educationalists in their efforts to find something which helps them to identify reflective capacity in individuals.

Mesirow (1981) sees levels (1) to (4) as characteristic of what he calls consciousness, and levels (5) to (7) as characteristic of critical consciousness. We do not know how much these are age related but it is worth remembering that Mesirow studied college returners who were presumably older women, to begin to develop his critical theory. Importantly, he relates critical consciousness and theoretical reflectivity to adult learning, therefore advocating the need to move towards perspective transformation in adult learning. Mesirow views perspective transformation as developing an understanding of 'reality' and thus developing a responsibility for decision-making, and this he believes is the essence of education. Of course, taking action following perspective transformation depends on the situation and our knowledge and skills as well as our personalities. Mesirow's work therefore makes the point that the relationship of reflection and change needs to be thoughtfully considered.

Table 9.3 Mesirow's levels of reflectivity. Adapted from Mesirow (1981).

(1) Reflectivity – awareness of a specific perception.
(2) Affective reflectivity – awareness of how we feel about the way we are perceiving, thinking or acting/habits.
(3) Discriminant Reflectivity – assessment of the efficacy of our perceptions, thoughts, actions, habits of doing things. Identifying immediate courses, recognising reality contexts and identifying our relationships in a situation.
(4) Judgemental reflectivity – making/becoming aware of value judgements about perceptions, thoughts, actions and habits.
(5) Conceptual reflectivity – self-reflection leading to questioning of values.
(6) Psychic reflection – recognition of the habit of making precipitant judgements on the basis of limited information. Recognising interests and anticipations influencing our perception, action and thinking.
(7) Theoretical reflection – awareness of reasons for our habit of precipitant judgement or conceptual inadequacy. Mesirow (1981) sees this last one as the process central to perspective transformation.

Goodman's theory of reflection

Goodman's (1984) theoretical ideas are based on his grounded theory work with student teachers, influenced by the work of Van Manen (1977) and Dewey (1933). Goodman (1984) distinguishes three levels of reflection (Table 9.4) that a reflective practitioner could achieve. These levels could serve as a broad guide for nurses and for teachers in assessing the quality and depth of reflective work.

Goodman makes the useful point that the focus of reflection needs to be clarified with students, otherwise it is all too easy to end up with most people focusing on the first level of reflection, as can be seen in some of the nursing research to date (see Chapter 1). While such theoretical work is useful in attempting to qualify people's reflection, Goodman himself makes the point that reflection is not merely a method of problem solving, but is a way of thinking and being, a point made by Sue Duke in Chapter 8. Goodman makes the link that reflection is about the

Table 9.4 The focus of reflection. Adapted from Goodman (1984).

1st level
Reflection to reach given objectives: Criteria for reflection are limited to technocratic issues of efficiency, effectiveness and accountability. The worth of objectives is taken for granted; reflection criteria are limited to accountability, efficiency and effectiveness. Students are concerned with what works, in maintaining the status quo.
2nd level
Reflection on the relationship between (nursing) principles and practice: There is an assessment of the implications and consequences of actions and beliefs as well as the underlying rationale for practice. A debate over principles and goals can be seen.
3rd level
Reflection which besides the above incorporates ethical and political concerns: Issues of justice, equality and emancipation enter deliberations over the value of professional goals and practice and the practitioner makes links between the setting of everyday practice and broader social structure and forces.

rational (e.g. organisation, selection, judgement and explanation) but also about the intuitive (e.g. imagination, emotions, insight, creativity and empathy). He also draws on Dewey's attitudes required for reflection, namely open-mindedness, responsibility and wholeheartedness. People who are open-minded take a look at rationales underlying what they initially might take for granted as right. They must also be motivated to 'synthesise ideas, make sense out of nonsense and apply information in an inspired direction' (p.20). Finally, people need the strength to face insecurities, fears, criticism and the upset of tradition in order to develop change; it is these things, says Goodman, that can get in the way of whole-heartedness. Thus courage to analyse and evaluate practice is also required.

Summarising a few key messages about frameworks for reflection

My experience tells me that the reflective cycle (Gibbs 1988) is particularly favoured by many undergraduate students, with the more complex frameworks often being adopted by higher degree students. The key factor seems to be finding something that helps you to get started and that eventually gives you the confidence to, as Bolton (2001) suggests, deconstruct your own practice.

All of the frameworks here have both their strengths and limitations and it is true to say that once again more research exploring their use in practice, both clinical and educational, would be welcome. Additionally, frameworks do not encompass all that reflection is or could be; you need to invest in developing the sorts of skills that Sue Atkins outlines in Chapter 2, think about the influences of coaching and facilitation on reflection, and generally have a look at the literature on reflection to get your own critical feel for it. Best of all you simply need to try it for yourself.

Exemplars from practice

The following exemplars from practice are contributions from a wide range of nurses and include both undergraduate and post-graduate work. These examples are presented as written by contributors, with pseudonyms for people and places as appropriate. For the first time I have included some examples that have been in previous editions of this book, rather than opting for a totally new set of exemplars. This is because there is a tendency for busy people to read only the latest edition of a book and consequently I have a feeling that a few very powerful exemplars of practice from past work do not get read that often. Also, I have found myself going back to some of these exemplars when I have been teaching and facilitating reflection myself, and so I make no apology for including them. Old and new, these exemplars simply serve to illustrate practitioners trying to reflect on their practice. Questions and pointers are also included in the text to encourage you to notice important things in the reflection which may help your own thinking and writing.

Exemplar 1

A final year undergraduate pre-registration student nurse reflecting on her community experience:

'A survey from Riverside Health Authority suggests that "75% of district nurses spend at least a quarter of their time treating leg ulcers" (Poulton 1991). I would suggest that the same applies to the district nurse I have been working with. I think the statement is incorrect in that the time is not spent simply on solely treating the leg ulcer. To simply treat an ulcer is probably ineffective and unhelpful for both patient and nurse. It is obvious in so many of the patients I have met that their needs far exceed the mere physical. Barry (who is 74 years old) lost his wife last year, he misses her very much. He has suffered with leg ulcers on and off for the past 30 years. They are presently being treated by the district nurses. Each time we have visited him he has been very pleased to see us and talks at length about what he has been doing recently. He always mentions his wife and describes his grief and his loneliness. It is in Barry's interest to continue his leg ulcer problem as it offers him an excuse for company from the district nurses who he gets on so well with. "Loneliness is a precipitating factor in many illnesses and in attention seeking behaviour. It is essential that psychological and social needs are recognised as such and not treated as medical problems" (Wise 1986).

If as a nurse I misunderstand the need for holistic care and find myself in a situation as described, I could see the patient as irresponsible for not adhering to the treatment I am offering for his leg ulcer. If, however, I can appreciate that Barry's loneliness is as great a problem as his leg ulcer, then I can begin to offer him the sort of care that he is looking for. I can avoid the personal frustration by accepting that being an effective practitioner is not merely about healing a leg ulcer, in this case it is also about healing a broken heart.'

- Take a look at this exemplar; is it easy to differentiate levels of reflection (see Goodman and Mesirow above) in this work?
- How are you affected by reading this account? What does it make you think about?
- How does this account make you feel?

Exemplar 2

A health visiting student evaluating her reflection on two challenging incidents from her practice and reviewing her personal learning:

'In this contract I have reflected on two unique incidents which I deemed to be challenging. I chose to reflect on a challenging situation because I thought I did not have the skills, knowledge, understanding or confidence to cope with these situations. Key features of learning I identified to help me cope with challenging situations were listening, empathy, adopting a non-judgemental approach and motivation.

Initially I didn't realise that these particular key features would enable me to understand how to cope with challenging situations. I began with searching for complex theories on coping strategies. However, through reflection, discussion with my practice teacher and reading literature, I realise that deeply understanding interpersonal skills was the key to helping me manage challenging situations. Realising why, when and how to listen to what clients were telling me as well as what they were not telling me, has enabled me to have a greater understanding of their feelings, thoughts and needs. I believe this is so important in my practice. Through understanding and listening to my clients I feel confident to provide an 'individual needs met' service. Instead of becoming nervous, feeling incompetent and concentrating on my own feelings, it is my intention to deeply listen to clients. As I gain understanding of their needs, this will empower me to cope with the situation.

I also now understand the real difference between sympathy and empathy and its importance in health visiting. This realisation helped me develop a whole new awareness of how to meet clients' needs. I now believe that being empathetic will enable me to portray to the client that I deeply understand them, their feelings, beliefs, values and thoughts. I think that if I can be empathetic towards my clients I am able to meet their deep rooted needs, instead of just superficially. I believe that sometimes it is also not necessary to take action or provide a resource to meet that need. Some clients do not want an answer to their problems, just a listener who acknowledges and understands them.

I also now feel competent to adopt a non-judgemental approach. This has stemmed from reflecting on my own beliefs, values and learnt behaviour. I have learnt that when you know yourself, not only can you change but you can also more easily accept other people's values and beliefs. I also feel more competent to assist my clients in motivation and bringing about behaviour change. This is through gaining theoretical understanding. Gaining theoretical knowledge will assist me in understanding what motivates my clients. This is also necessary in understanding what motivates myself. If I am aware of what motivates me, I will be able to help others more clearly (Kagan *et al.* 1986).

Reflecting on myself has been a soul searching experience in which I have learnt a lot about myself. The honesty of my reflection has been somewhat eye opening. I thought it was important to be honest with myself in order to truly reflect. It was difficult being honest with myself. I had to look deep into my soul and reflect on all my beliefs and values which make me what I am. I also found it trying at times because I had to be honest with my practice teacher. Being honest with myself was one thing, allowing myself to be honest with someone else was very difficult. However working with my practice teacher proved to be very valuable. She guided me on the right path and drew out thoughts and behaviours that I might not have addressed on my own. My practice teacher also challenged me and this has allowed me to look at new ways of working and take my practice forward.

I now feel I have the knowledge, skills and understanding to cope with situations I once deemed challenging. Although I think I will always come across some challenging situations they will appear to be challenging for different reasons. Learning how to cope with these situations will be ongoing. I do realise that I will never achieve total self-awareness, but I can work at making constructive use out of my experiences throughout life in order to enhance my relationships and make more use of my interpersonal skills (Kagan *et al.* 1986). I also believe that learning about oneself as a person and as a practitioner is an evolving process which develops with time and experience.'

- What do you think about this student's judgement and evaluation about her health visiting experiences?
- Have a look at the issues that arise for the student in making the decision to communicate honestly about her practice. How will you handle this decision in your own work?

Exemplar 3

Written by a post-registration diploma student working in a critical care setting. Here she reflects on the issues connected with body image while caring for a women recovering from multiple injuries:

'I get up in the morning and look in the mirror and I have to say, am not usually happy with what I see. Too fat, too spotty, grey hair, the list could be endless. This shows that I, on occasion, have a problem with my body image. Schilder (1935) cited in Price (1990) defines body image as the picture of our body that we form in our mind; the way our body appears to ourselves. Simply put then, body image is the way we see ourselves. Perhaps I am unhappy with my body image, because obviously it evolves throughout life? Cronan (1993) suggests that body image problems arise naturally within the aging process because of conflicts between feelings and looks. I still feel inside a lot of the time as I did at 22, 23 – same moral values, beliefs, sense of fun – so I feel young but I look every day at my 29 years – what a conflict. Society also puts pressure on your body image, for example you only have to look at the media to see that good-looking equals thin. Where is the room for the world's fat, birth-marked and teeth-braced people? Salter (1988) agrees, suggesting that society exerts great pressure on us to comply with a certain image. While Cronan specifies fashion, mass media, and socialisation and peer pressure as factors affecting body image formation, I have problems accepting my body image which is 'normal', but will this knowledge help me address the problems of people with altered body image?'

- What feel do you get for this practitioner's sense of self-awareness?

'What is altered body image? Wright (1986) suggests that any change in appearance or function of any part of our body threatens our body image. This change does not have to be obvious scarring or disfigurement. This is why I have chosen this objective. Every patient on the unit will have experienced some change in function that will affect how they feel about themselves. I want to develop an insight into what I can do to help and assist them come to terms with this change.

K was a 40-year-old lady who had been admitted to the ward with multiple injuries from ITU. All her injuries were fixed but she required split skin grafts to her left leg… As K's condition improved she became aware of the physical aspect of altered body image. Dewing (1989) suggests that body image is composed of two components – the physical and the psychological. As will be revealed, K had many psychological barriers to acceptance of her physical disabilities. Awareness of the skin grafts came only the first time they were dressed. When I began to take the dressings down, I explained that the grafts would look very red and raw, and that if she didn't want to look at them that was OK. I had spent a few days building up trust and gaining a rapport before this. I felt that if K trusted me she would be able to cope better; that was why I explained that her sites would not seem 'good' from her point of view but would probably look healthy and good from mine. Gaster (1995) suggests that if the key characteristic in professionals' relations with clients is trust, the key values are integrity and fair conduct. I had not wanted to give K an unrealistic view of what her leg would look like. K was devastated – pavement pizza, raw meat, were adjectives that she used. I spent a long time with her while she cried, looking back grieving for what she had lost. I tried to reiterate that things would improve and that her leg would not look like that forever. Piff (1986) suggests that the reaction that patients receive to their disfigurement strongly influences how they cope in the future. I am pleased that I am aware of this – after 7 years not much of what I see can shock me – but I must help to prepare more junior staff to mask any adverse reactions that they may have.'

- How do you think this nurse's use of the literature has helped in her reflection?

'A few days later one of our old patients was readmitted who had massive skin grafts to his leg that he had received six months previously. I asked him if he would mind showing his leg to K, and he agreed. Kim did seem happier knowing that cosmetically the site on her leg would improve. Drench (1994) states that interaction with people who have similar body image deficits but lead active lives seems to help the person make the transition to a new and satisfactory body image. I thought that I was beginning to make headway with K but she remained very emotionally labile – one moment happy, the next sobbing uncontrollably. I spent a lot of time with K, listening and talking. I felt that I had built a good trusting relationship at last. Trust, according to MacGinley (1993), being very important if a nurse is to help a patient adapt to an altered body image...

   I thought we were doing a good job of promoting acceptance by K of her altered body image, but she was continually very emotional, crying with no seeming end. We tried to get her to see a counsellor to help her psychologically to come to terms with her injury, but she would not. I was beginning to get worn out – you can only give so much. When K cried now I found it difficult to empathise. I was beginning to get very judgemental, i.e. thinking why doesn't she pull herself together! I haven't got time for this. MacGinley suggests that the nurse should be able to empathisise with her patient's feelings, e.g. anger, depression, in a positive accepting manner without being judgemental. I was no longer able to do this. I found it difficult to care for K. Trying to deal with her strong feeling of despair and anger became difficult and occupied more and more time, until sometimes I left her to cry because it was just too much for me to take. On reflection I should have arranged not to look after her for a few shifts, I should have negotiated a change to give myself a break.'

- How easy do you think it is for a nurse to admit these sorts of feelings?
- How would you feel about sharing similar experiences with a mentor or supervisor?

Exemplar 4

An undergraduate student reflecting on the basic tasks of physical caring on a medical ward:

> 'This particularly frail and emaciated 86-year-old gentleman presented with digoxin toxicity. He also suffered from progressive cardiac failure, osteoarthritis and bilateral cataracts. Observing this gentleman's unsuccessful attempts to manipulate cutlery and manoeuvre food to his mouth before finally pushing aside the uneaten meal was a sobering lesson. Had I inadvertently contributed, albeit in a minor and unobtrusive manner, to the endemic of hospital-induced malnutrition? Although conscientiously providing a high density diet to compensate for his meagre appetite, enthusiastically encouraging him to eat smaller quantities frequently and arranging every conceivable need within his grasp, I had nonetheless neglected the simple mechanics of the process. To his arthritic hands a sealed dessert represented an impenetrable barrier: an additional and unnecessary frustration for him and food for thought indeed.'

- At what point on the reflective cycle (see Gibbs 1988) would you identify the above?

> 'The most obvious solution also seemed the least desirable. Would feeding this gentleman preserve his self-esteem or be interpreted as a humiliating and undignified insult, a further unwelcome confirmation of his increasing disability? Was it necessary to compromise his sensibilities in order to ensure he ate enough?
>
> Planning with him an acceptable diet revealed additional problems. The size of meals posed an uninviting ordeal sufficient to dampen his appetite. An impaired ability to smell, taste and see food deprived him of the stimulus to eat; pain and hunger were experienced as similar and frequently confused sensations. Although equipped with complete dentures chewing was both arduous and exhausting. The three-meal-a-day hospital regimen was dissimilar from his accustomed habit. The embarrassment of constipation and of faecal incontinence was incentive enough to avoid eating.
>
> I endeavoured to forewarn him of an impending meal and prior to its arrival, encouraged him to visualise its contents in an attempt to whet his appetite; a mint aperitif refreshed his mouth and stimulated gastric motility. I adjusted his position, tucked a napkin onto his chest and arranged his food in a clock face to assist him to locate each mouthful. Broad handled utensils and gentle coaxing compensated for his lack of dexterity. A small semi-liquid and strong flavoured meal, supplemented by between-meal snacks, proved more palatable and manageable. Replenishing a beaker of fruit juice and inviting him to use a drinking straw provided readily accessible fluid.'

- Has the student's reflection moved on through the reflective cycle to a different point?

'Sharing and resolving the eating problems encountered by this gentleman demonstrate, I believe, a genuine concern for his well-being and contributed to some small degree toward rejuvenating his diminished sense of personal effectiveness and self-worth.'

- How easy do you find it to communicate the seemingly everyday things about your practice?
- How often do you reflect on your usual everyday practice? Could you make the reflective effort to give it a go? Do you think you would learn anything from it?

Exemplar 5

Two extracts from a student health visitor's reflective learning contract. As an experienced hospital nurse she reflects on the issues and challenges that confront her as a novice in the community setting:

'Working in the community is in sharp contrast to working within a hospital environment. I have little experience of this aspect of nursing and initially I felt the skills I had could not easily be transferred into it. Cain (1995) suggests that community nursing is the same as hospital nursing; the skills are simply transferred to a different setting. This was not my personal experience and in my first term I felt anxious, apprehensive and deskilled and wondered whether these skills could be transferred. Mackenzie (1990) suggests that far from the hospital skills being easily transferred there are differences that actively work against such transformation. A key example is the fact that community nursing is client-led and controlled, whereas the opposite is true of hospital life. It could be said that for nursing care to be therapeutic there needs to be positive inter-action and communication between the nurse and the client, as people. This is in contrast to the work of Byrne and Heyman (1997). In their qualitative study of A and E nurses' perceptions of caring, while nurses acknowledged the need for psychological support, they felt there was no time for such care. The emphasis was on keeping the patients moving and the department running, and as such was seen as more important than psychological care. Working in someone's home requires skills that do not imply a lack of time and an emphasis to keep things moving. Of course, attention has to be paid to the management of time, but experience is beginning to show me that this too is client-led in the com-munity.'

- What resources is this practitioner using to critically examine her first experi-ences of working in the community?

'One particular incident occurred very early on while I was in practice. Penny, my practice teacher, was taking a post-natal group. I found myself alone in the clinic kitchen with a very weepy and depressed mother. She was pouring out her heart to me. I felt awkward and didn't know what to say to her, wondering what advice I would give.'

- Where would you put the above on the reflective cycle (Gibbs 1988)?

'This was in contrast to my previous job where I felt confident and qualified to give advice. She was crying throughout the time; although I wanted to put my arms around her to comfort her, I did not know this lady and it didn't seem "right". Putting my arms around her may have had the effect of stopping her talking and I didn't want to do that; I stood beside her and listened. During this incident I didn't speak for some time. This seemed intuitively to be the right thing to do and I let her continue. She continued with many feelings about the baby, he was so good, he was this, he was that... etc. I felt I had to interject, although I was feeling nervous. I said to her, "It's not about the baby, it's about how you are feeling." She thought herself a bad mother, she wasn't breast feeding, good mothers breast feed, she was ashamed that with everything – a good home, no financial worries and a supportive partner – that she could feel like this and it had all been a big mistake.

Expectations on today's mothers are immense; the pressure to be beautiful, intelligent, hold down a good job and then when the time is right have a baby. Glossy magazines imply the baby will also fall into the beautiful, intelligent and will sleep all night category. Lydia was all of these things and yet here she was crying in the kitchen. How different reality is. During this time I was actively thinking she may be suffering from post-natal depression or maybe she was just having an off day, but with little first hand experience of this I didn't want to jump in and label her.'

- Where do you think the above paragraph would fit on the reflective cycle?

'Reflection is initiated by an awareness of uncomfortable feelings and thoughts, which arise from the realisation that the knowledge one was applying in a situation was not itself sufficient to explain what was happening in that unique situation. I did feel uncomfortable but on reflection I would change very little. I learnt that actively listening and not talking are therapeutic. As my confidence as a health visitor increases so does my ability to recognise in myself my strengths and weaknesses. I considered whether Lydia had really been listened to in the past. It may have been her perception that health professionals had a role to play and with all her obvious support, that any anxieties must be superficial. This demonstrates how important it is not to be judgemental when meeting clients and is something I will value for future practice.

When Lydia was ready to go she turned to me and said "thank you for listening". I was not expecting this and was quite surprised more by the "for listening" than for the "thank you". Why was I surprised? Melia (1987) discusses the occupational socialisation of nurses in which they learn the unwritten rules of the occupational setting. This included the concept that talking was not working and the need for nursing staff to look busy. The nature of workplace socialisation is further outlined by Smith (1992) who suggested that at the severe end, nurse socialisation turned an emotionally attuned student into a cynical practitioner preoccupied with "real" nursing tasks. I considered the A and E environment; as someone often in charge in A and E the pressure to keep the flow of patients moving through the department is intense and challenging;

s research to suggest that this pressure can result in less effective care for
ts (Byrne & Heyman 1997). Looking back, with some 150 plus people
ng the department per day, it was not surprising that time was the enemy
of effective nursing care. This incident has affected my practice as it has
demonstrated to me the difference in dealing with emotional rather than purely
physical conditions, and has highlighted where my skills are transferable and
where they need further development.'

● Take a look at Stephenson's framework for reflection. Can you see elements of
  her framework in the exemplar above?

Exemplar 6

Extracts from a nurse's diary. These are snippets of reflective observation that were
not written for an assessment but simply to express the author's experiences in
writing, in an attempt to reflect on her experiences in practice:

'I looked after an 89-year-old lady who had had major surgery. She was left with
a wound that was difficult to heal and she had severe arthritis. She was very
weak and frail but cognitively "with it". The ward was very busy and there was
little time to really sit down and check through the total needs for a lady like this.
  For good wound healing a person must logically have good nutrition. I
watched this lady; she ate small portions, did not have a good appetite and
found it difficult to feed herself because of her arthritis and sheer weakness. I
had to help her a great deal at lunch time. She needed more independence! She
had some thick-handled cutlery that her sister had brought in, but I discovered
that it was left-handed and her dominant side was right, making eating even
more difficult.
  I protected her clothing, helped her to sit more upright, got some ordinary
cutlery and discreetly helped her with her meal. I found some Build-Up drinks
and explained briefly about nutrition and wound healing; she understood the
logic well enough. Later I referred her to the dietician and to the occupational
therapist in the hope that we could improve her nutritional intake and optimise
what she did eat with a high calorie, high protein diet and also help her to eat
more independently with the correct equipment.
  It strikes me that full assessment of the older person can be a difficult thing to
achieve, particularly in acute wards where the emphasis is on the acute phase of
illness. This experience reassures me that teaching students the importance of
good nutrition in the older person is vital in order to give them knowledge from
which to start building their assessment and planning skills.'

'I spent some time talking with a lady who had just had pelvic floor surgery. She
described her problem before surgery, how her GP had not offered any solution
to her incontinence and how when she swung a golf club, urine would escape
from her bladder; she described further indignities caused by the incontinence.
She changed GP and was then referred for surgery. Her new GP was horrified
(so was I) that the previous one had done little to help. She said "I mentioned it

when I went along with another problem." I was horrified to think that she had put up with such appalling symptoms for so long. She said "Sometimes it was so bad I had blisters down my thighs", "I worried about smelling."

This really made me think about how dependent people are on skilled primary health care, which relies on effective diagnosis and referral. I am still left wondering why a GP would simply do nothing! Didn't he or she pick up on any cues during consultation? Could he or she really be unaware of treatment possibilities? On talking with this lady it was also apparent that taboo subjects such as this do not get talked about, therefore maybe many people feel they are the only ones with this sort of problem. I was glad I had got into conversation; it gave me a little more insight than just looking in a textbook to find out more about pelvic floor surgery, and it reasserts my belief that effective communication is a key factor in good nursing and good medicine.

Any surgery has its difficulties and is not to be taken lightly, but I had a real sense that this lady has also been given new hope for her golf, swimming and everything, and just generally not having to worry about embarrassing herself in public.'

- Take a look at these diary entries once you have read Melanie Jasper's chapter on journal and diary keeping (Chapter 5). Can you identify the feelings that emerge from these snippets of writing? How could you improve the critical analysis above? What do you think that the nurse has learnt from these experiences?

Conclusion

I hope this final chapter serves as a useful reference point when beginning your journey into using reflection or in helping others to do so, and also that the reflective exemplars have given you some insight into other people's writing. I believe that they provide narrative evidence that nurses can use the power of storytelling to unearth what nursing is about, and that the process of reflection can encourage and capture analytical thinking and open-mindedness about practice, as well as a willingness and ability to influence things for the better. There are always things that writing does not capture; it is not possible to show the development of reflection through a few exemplars, or reveal all the contextual information that enables practitioners to reflect on their experiences. These are things that you need to experience and think about for yourself with support from facilitators, teachers and colleagues.

Acknowledgement

My sincere thanks to all those enthusiastic practitioners who were willing to share their reflective work with others.

nces

    '. & Schön, D. (1974) *Theory in Practice*. Jossey Bass, San Francisco.
Atkins, S. & Murphy, C. (1993) Reflection: a review of the literature. *Journal of Advanced Nursing*, **18**(8), 1188–92.
Bolton, G. (2001) *Reflective Practice. Writing and Professional Development*. Paul Chapman Publishing Ltd, London.
Boud, D., Keogh, R. & Walker, D. (1985) *Reflection: Turning learning into experience*. Kogan Page, London.
Brockbank, A. & McGill, I. (1998) *Facilitating Reflective Learning in Higher Education*. Society for Research in Higher Education and OU Press, Buckingham.
Burnard, P. (1991) Improving through reflection. *Journal of District Nursing*, May, 10–12.
Burns, S. & Bulman, C. (eds) (2000) *Reflective Practice. The Growth of the Professional Practitioner*, 2nd edn. Blackwell Science, Oxford.
Burton, A.J. (2000) Reflection: nursing's practice and education panacea? *Journal of Advanced Nursing*, **31**(5), 1009–17.
Byrne, G. & Heyman, R. (1997) Understanding nurses' communication with patients in A and E departments using a symbolic interactionist perspective. *Journal of Advanced Nursing*, **26**, 93–100.
Cain, P. (1995) *Community Nursing. Dimensions and Dilemmas*. Arnold, London.
Carr, E.C.J. (1996) Reflecting on clinical practice: hectoring talk or reality. *Journal of Clinical Nursing*, **5**, 289–95.
Clarke, M. (1986) Action and reflection: practice and theory in nursing. *Journal of Advanced Nursing*, **11**, 3–11.
Clinton, M. (1998) On reflection in action: unaddressed issues in refocusing the debate in reflective practice. *International Journal of Nursing Practice*, **4**(30), 197–203.
Cotton, A. (2001) Private thoughts in public spheres; issues in reflection and reflective practices in nursing. *Journal of Advanced Nursing*, **36**(4), 512–19.
Cronan, L. (1993) Management of the patient with altered body image. *British Journal of Nursing*, **2**(5), 257–61.
Cullingford, S. (1991) Learning from experience. *Senior Nurse* **11**(6), 25–8.
Day, C. (1993) Reflection: a necessary but not sufficient condition for professional development. *British Educational Research Journal*, **19**(1), 83–93.
Dewing, J. (1989) Altered body image. *Surgical Nurse*, **2**(4), 17–20.
Dewey, J. (1933) *How We Think. A restatement of the relation of reflective thinking to the educative process*. DC Heath, Massachusetts.
Drench, M. (1994) Changes in body image secondary to disease. *Rehabilitation Nursing*, **19**(1), 31–6.
Driscoll, J. (1994) Reflective practice for practise. *Senior Nurse*, **13**(7), 47–50.
Eraut, M. (1994) *Developing Professional Knowledge and Competence*. The Falmer Press, London.
Friere, P. (1972) *Pedagogy of the Oppressed*. Herder and Herder, New York.
Gaster, L. (1995) *Quality in Public Services. Managers Choice*. Open University Press, Buckingham.
Ghaye, T. & Lilyman, S. (1997) *Learning journals and critical incidents: Reflective practice for health care professionals*. Quay Books, London.
Ghaye, T. & Lilyman, S. (2000) *Reflection: Principles and practice for healthcare professionals*. Mark Allen Publishing Ltd, London.
Gibbs, G. (1988) *Learning by Doing. A Guide to Teaching and Learning Methods*. Oxford Polytechnic, Oxford.

Goodman, J. (1984) Reflection and teacher education: A case study and theoretical analysis. *Interchange*, 15(3), 9–26.

Greenwood, J. (1993a) Reflective practice: a critique of the work of Argyris and Schön. *Journal of Advanced Nursing*, 18, 1183–7.

Greenwood, J. (1993b) Some considerations concerning practice and feedback in nursing education. *Journal of Advanced Nursing*, 18, 1999–2002.

Greenwood, J. (1998) The role of reflection in single and double loop learning. *Journal of Advanced Nursing*, 27, 1048–53.

Hargreaves, J. (1997) Using patients: exploring the ethical dimension of reflective practice in nurse education. *Journal of Advanced Nursing*, 25, 223–38.

Heath, H. (1998) Paradigm dialogues and dogma: finding a place for research, nursing models and reflective practice. *Journal of Advanced Nursing*, 28(2), 288–94.

James, C.R. & Clarke, B.A. (1994) Reflective practice in nursing: issues and implications for nursing education. *Nurse Education Today*, 14, 82–90.

Jarvis, P. (1992) Reflective practice and nursing. *Nurse Education Today*, 12, 174–81.

Jarvis, P. & Gibson, S. (eds) (1997) *The Teacher, Practitioner and Mentor in Nursing, Midwifery, Health Visiting and the Social Services*, 2nd edn. Stanley Thornes, Cheltenham.

Jay, J.K. & Johnson, K.L. (2002) Capturing complexity: a typology of reflective practice for teacher education. *Teaching and Teacher Education*, 18, 73–85.

Johns, C. (1993) Professional supervision. *Journal of Nursing Management*, 1, 9–18.

Johns, C. (1994) Guided reflection. In: *Reflective Practice in Nursing. The Growth of the Professional Practitioner* (eds A. Palmer, S. Burns & C. Bulman). Blackwell Science, Oxford.

Johns, C. (1995a) The value of reflective practice for nursing *Journal of Clinical Nursing*, 4, 23–30.

Johns, C. (1995b) Framing learning through reflection within Carper's fundamental ways of knowing in nursing. *Journal of Advanced Nursing*, 22, 226–34.

Johns, C. (2000) *Becoming a Reflective Practitioner. A reflective and holistic approach to clinical nursing, practice development and clinical supervision*. Blackwell Science, Oxford.

Johns, C. & Freshwater, D. (1998) *Transforming Nursing Through Reflective Practice*. Blackwell Science, Oxford.

Kagan, C., Evans, J. & Kay, B. (1986) *A Manual of Interpersonal Skills for Nurses*. Harper and Row, London.

Kim, H.S. (1999) Critical reflective inquiry for knowledge development in nursing practice. *Journal of Advanced Nursing*, 29(50), 1205–12.

MacGinley, K.J. (1993) Nursing care of the patient with altered body image. *British Journal of Nursing*, 2(22), 1098–102.

Mackenzie, A. (1990) *Learning from experience in the community – an ethnographic study of district nurse*. PhD thesis, University of Surrey.

Mackintosh, C. (1998) Reflection: a flawed strategy for the nursing profession. *Nurse Education Today*, 18, 553–7.

Mallik, M. (1998) The role of nurse educators in the development of reflective practitioners: a selective case study of the Australian and UK experience. *Nurse Education Today*, 18, 52–63.

Melia, K. (1987) *Learning and Working. The Occupational Socialisation of Nurses*. Tavistock, London.

Mesirow, J. (1981) A critical theory of adult learning and education. *Adult Education*, 32(1), 3–24.

Newell, R. (1992) Anxiety, accuracy and reflection: the limits of professional development. *Journal of Advanced Nursing*, 17, 1326–33.

Piff, C. (1986) Facing Up to Disfigurement. *Nursing Times*, 82, 16–17.

Poulton, B. (1991) Factors influencing patient compliance. *Nursing Standard Supplement,* 12, 5, (5).

Price, B. (1990) *Body Image: Nursing Concepts and Care.* Prentice Hall, London.

Reid, B. (1993) 'But we're doing it already!' Exploring a response to the concept of reflective practice in order to improve its facilitation. *Nurse Education Today,* 13, 305–9.

Richardson, R. (1995) Humpty Dumpty: reflection and reflective nursing practice. *Journal of Advanced Nursing,* 21, 1044–50.

Rolfe, G., Freshwater, D. & Jasper, M. (2001) *Critical Reflection for Nursing and the Helping Professions; a User's Guide.* Palgrave Macmillan, London.

Salter, M. (1988) *Altered Body Image: The Nurses Role.* John Wiley and Sons, Chichester.

Saylor, C.R. (1990) Reflection and professional education: art, science and competency. *Nurse Education,* 15(2), 8–11.

Scanlan, J.M. & Chernomas, W.M. (1997) Developing the reflective teacher. *Journal of Advanced Nursing,* 25, 1138–43.

Schön, D.A. (1983) *The Reflective Practitioner.* Basic Books. Harper Collins, San Francisco.

Schön, D.A. (1987) *Educating the Reflective Practitioner.* Jossey Bass, San Francisco.

Smith P. (1992) *The Emotional Labour of Nursing. How Nurses Care.* Macmillan Education, Basingstoke.

Stephenson, S. (2000) Exemplars of reflection. In: *Reflective Practice in Nursing. The Growth of the Professional Practitioner* (eds S. Burns & C. Bulman). Blackwell Science, Oxford.

Street, A. (1991) *From Image to Action: Reflection in Nursing Practice.* Deakin University Press, Geelong.

Van Manen, M. (1977) Linking ways of knowing with ways of being practical. *Curriculum Inquiry,* 6(3), 205–28.

Wise, G. (1986) Overcoming loneliness. *Nursing Times,* 28, 37–42.

Wong, F.K.Y., Loke, A.Y.L., Wong, M., Tse, H., Kan, E. & Kember, D. (1997) An action research study into the development of nurses as reflective practitioners. *Journal of Nursing Education,* 36(10), 476–81.

Wright, B. (1986) *Caring in Crisis.* Churchill Livingstone, London.

Index